Decoding Pelvic Pain

Lavonne Pineda, DC

LCP MEDIA

DISCLAIMER: This book is not about treating disease, and no information contained in it should be construed as such. This book is intended as a reference manual only, not as a medical manual. The information presented here is designed to help you make informed decisions about your health. It is not intended as a substitute for any treatment that may have been prescribed by your doctor, who is acquainted with your specific needs. This book should be used as a supplement rather than replace the advice of your doctor or other trained health professional. If you suspect you have a medical problem, please seek competent medical care. All efforts have been made to assure the accuracy of the information contained in this book as of the date of publication. This publisher and author disclaim liability for any medical outcomes that may occur as a result of applying the methods suggested in this book. Some of the names and identifying characteristics of the individuals discussed in this book have been changed to protect their privacy.

Published by LCP Media Group, San Jose, California (408) 448-4070

LCP Media may be purchased for educational, business, or sales promotional use. For information, please email info@pelvicpainprogram.com

Without limiting the rights under copyright reserved above, no part of this publication may be reproduced, stored in, or introduced into a retrieval system, or transmitted, in any form or by any means (electronic, mechanical, photocopying, recording, or otherwise), without prior written permission of both the copyright owner and the above publisher of this book. Excerpts or quotations are allowed for a book review.

First Edition, Printed in USA
Illustrations by Austin Knop
Copyright © 2018 by Dr. Lavonne Pineda
ISBN-13: 9781793951656

Table of Contents

Chapter 1	Introduction to Pelvic Pain	1
Chapter 2	Dr. P's Philosophy	9
Chapter 3	Dr. P's Pelvic Pain Program (P4)	17
Chapter 4	Restore the Floor Beginning Pain Relief	21
Chapter 5	Preventing Flare-Ups	33
Chapter 6	Gut Health	37
Chapter 7	Pain Relief Naturally!	45
Chapter 8	Taking Back Your Power	79
Chapter 9	Strengthening and Stretching	88
Chapter 10	Now you Know!	98
Chapter 11	Bonus: Pelvic Anti-Inflammatory Diet Sample Recipes	100
Bibliography		125

Acknowledgments

There are so many people who have supported me during this process. Without them, this book couldn't have happened. First and foremost, my wife. She was there throughout my journey, both in getting to the other side of chronic pain, and in writing this book. I am very grateful for her constant belief in me and for encouraging me to never give up. Dr. Jeri Anderson, DC, a mentor, and friend, who has always been there for me. Dr. Edward Cremata, DC, RN, who pushed me toward a career as a chiropractor, and most recently, for helping get my body and mind to the next level in healing. Dr. Dana Grenman, DC for her incredible skills with trigger points and Pelvic Floor Dysfunction. Peter Riggio for his expertise in cannabinoids, and for answering my endless questions. Patty Dominguez for her humor and unfailing enthusiasm and guidance, at any time of the day or night! Lastly, Austin Knop for his amazing illustrations of trigger points and anatomy.

A Note from Dr. Pineda

I have been in the health field for over 29 years. My greatest joy has been the ability to witness a quality of life change in people. I had never considered writing a book as part of this mission. That was, until I experienced chronic pain. It was then that I realized I needed a new, integrated, approach to my own health.

I was in severe, constant pain, and willing to try anything. Many of those modalities didn't work or made my pain worse. Desperation pushed me to research answers to heal and get my life back. It was then I felt a huge responsibility to share this journey in the hopes it could help you move from desperation to hope too. This book will walk you through the basics of chronic pelvic pain and why you continue to get flare-ups, and then move into the solution, so you too can begin your journey of pain and symptom relief.

Yours in health,

Dr. Lavonne

Chapter 1

Introduction to Pelvic Pain

I'm Dr. Pineda (Dr P), Chronic Pelvic Pain is personal for me, and a problem for men and women everywhere. Yet not much is known about it. How is it that pelvic pain is a serious problem, and we don't know much about it? Research shows that approximately 1 in 7 women will end up suffering Chronic Pelvic Pain, also known as CPP[1]. One study in primary care practices showed 39% of reproductive-aged women suffered pelvic pain[2]. 10% of all referrals to gynecologists is for pelvic pain[3]. Those are high numbers; the odds are many of us will go through it at some point in our lives. Pelvic pain isn't specific to women, men can suffer pain in the pelvic area too, although compared to women, occurrence of CPP in men is so much lower that pelvic pain is often seen as something only women suffer from. (Lucky us!)

So, what really is pelvic pain? What causes it? How can you try to overcome it? What are the solutions to help you, if you unfortunately are (or when you become) a victim? I talk about all this, and more, in this book.

---

[1] (Mathias, Kuppermann, Liberman, Lipschutz, & Steege, 1996)
[2] (Jamieson & Steege, 1996)
[3] (Reiter, 1990)

What is Pelvic Pain?

Before I can explain what chronic pelvic pain is, I must first discuss the pelvis. The pelvis is the lowest part of the abdomen in the human body. Since pelvic pain is something that affects more women than men, the information in this book focuses on women. If you have questions about pelvic pain in men, please send me an email.

The pelvis houses some very important organs, including the bowel, bladder, womb or uterus, and the ovaries. Pelvic pain is discomfort you experience in this region of your body. It may originate from any of the pelvic housed organs, or nearby muscles, blood vessels, or the joints.

It's a persistent pain that just won't go away. You have probably experienced pelvic pain at some point in your life, but unless it has been recurring in nature, or is something that you haven't been able to get rid of, you don't need to worry. Why? Because short term or one-time pain is **acute pelvic pain** which should resolve itself in under three months (or so). What we are talking about is long term pain, or chronic pain. This is pain that persists or recurs on a regular basis - it doesn't go away on its own, like acute pain usually does.

Chronic pain is consistent, and it has probably been troubling you for some time now. Doctors usually classify pain as chronic if it lasts for three to six months, or longer. Therefore, if you or someone you know have pelvic pain that has persisted for months, it is likely Chronic Pelvic Pain.

In women, pelvic pain is a symptom of an issue in the reproductive, urinary or digestive systems, or it is from musculoskeletal sources. The intensity of the pain depends on the source. It can be dull or sharp; constant or intermittent; mild, moderate or severe. But the issue may not stop there. You may experience other problems too. The pain can spread to your lower back, buttocks (like it did for me), or thighs, causing even more discomfort. The spread of pain to other areas is often caused by the development of trigger points. When pain levels increase, the pelvic floor goes into an increased 'tone' state. This is when your body naturally goes into a guarded state (clenching). This is the body's natural survival instinct to protect the area from any more harm. Some people experience pelvic pain only at certain times, or only during certain activities, such as urination, or sexual activity.

Meet my patient Marianne. Marianne started experiencing low back and pelvic pain after receiving a deep Thai Massage. Her pain progressively got worse, until she had constant sharp pain, with burning, tingling, and numbness down her legs. She sought care from her medical doctor who took x-rays of her low back and prescribed pharmaceuticals (a type of benzo and opiate). The pain continued, so she was referred for an MRI of the lumbar spine. The MRI showed degeneration, and disk herniations at two levels. She then went to an acupuncturist, seeking relief. That evening, her pain got so bad she went to the hospital emergency room (ER). There she was given an injection of morphine and sent home with another, more addicting, opiate. Her doctor then referred her to a pain management doctor to manage her pain levels.

Marianne came to my office three days after being given morphine from the ER physician. She was desperate. She didn't want to have to take opioids in order to function. I could see she was in extreme pain just filling out the paperwork. She could not sit for more than 20 minutes. Lying down, and standing, caused her extreme pain. She could not lift anything without increasing pain levels. Driving was difficult due to prolonged sitting. She was sleeping less than three hours a night. Climbing stairs was difficult. Tying her shoes was a painful chore.

While taking her history, she let me know she is self-employed. She owns two thriving esthetician businesses, in two cities, requiring her to travel between both and her home. She is the sole practitioner, running both of them. In her current condition, she had to shut them both down for a month. This was adding to her stress levels.

Her x-rays showed that her pelvis was rotated, and she had lumbar spine arthritis. Her MRI results showed several areas of concern. After examining her, and evaluating her x-rays, it was obvious she had dysfunction in her pelvis. I gave her a chiropractic adjustment of her pelvis. She got up and burst into tears of relief. It was the first time in five months that Marianne had relief from the constant pain.

When she returned the next day, I was able to adjust her again and start her on a program to alleviate pain in her pelvis. I sent her home with breathing exercises to start. When she returned the next week, her pain levels were greatly reduced, and she was smiling. After two weeks of home breathing exercises, and chiropractic care, she was able to return to work. Once the pain levels decreased for Marianne, we were able to identify the physiological patterns she had adopted, which had contributed to her pain for years. She has been doing amazingly well doing all of her home exercises, and she continues to improve. She went back to running her business full time, with minimal residual pain. Marianne told me her goal for this program has shifted. It is not about pain relief any longer but being better than she was before she felt the pain.

What Causes Pelvic Pain?

The causes of pelvic pain for men and women are too many to count. In this book, I discuss the more common ones.

Chronic Pelvic Pain (CPP)

As I've shared with you already, pelvic pain that has lasted for more than six months is called Chronic Pelvic Pain (CPP)[4] and show 1 in every 7 women might suffer from CPP[5]. The cause of the pain is sometimes readily identifiable, and sometimes it remains hidden for a while. Often it is difficult to accurately pinpoint the cause and source of CPP. Depression, chronic stress, and a past history of sexual or physical abuse, increase the risk of developing chronic pelvic pain. Emotional stress, and distress, often worsens pain, causing further emotional distress.

Here are some other causes of pelvic pain for men and women. This list is not exhaustive:

- Endometriosis
- Bowel or bladder problems
- Appendicitis
- Irritable Bowel Syndrome (IBS)
- Cystitis
- Colitis
- Adhesions
- Strangulated Hernia
- Muscle and Bone Problems

---

[4] (Singh, MD, 2018)
[5] (Mathias, Kuppermann, Liberman, Lipschutz, & Steege, 1996)

- Pelvic Inflammatory Disease (PID)
- Fibromyalgia
- Colon Cancer
- Kidney Stones
- Intestinal Obstruction
- Urinary Tract Infection (UTI)
- Prostatitis
- Chronic constipation
- Chronic (nonbacterial) Prostatitis
- Chronic Orchalgia
- Prostatodynia

With so many potential underlying causes of pelvic pain, the challenge becomes how to treat pelvic pain. Medical doctors search for the cause, which may be one of the above, or not, and treat that. The pelvic pain is less of a concern to them. You may find yourself on medication for IBS, but still in a tremendous amount of pain. Pelvic pain is very misunderstood and poorly managed. You may be sent from specialist to specialist, with no relief. The cause of your chronic pelvic pain remaining unclear. This is extremely frustrating (I know! I was there!)

Meet Lydia. Lydia was lifting a large, heavy, pot off the counter. She was twisting and heard a pop. Immediately she experienced sharp low back and leg pain. She waited three days thinking it would go away. The pain got so bad she went to the ER. The doctor told her it was probably a herniated disc. He prescribed medication and told her to go home and ice her back.

Lydia has been a self-employed house cleaner for many years. She was unable to work due to the extreme pain. She could not sit for long periods, so driving was painful. She couldn't bend, lift, twist, or climb stairs - all activities she had to do to work. She couldn't sleep through the night.

I had seen Lydia before, so I was familiar with her history. She works very hard. Lydia is someone who will work through her pain, to keep working. She has a petite frame which makes many of her work tasks, like lifting vacuums, challenging. The physical demands of her job are tough on her body.

When she came to my office I noticed that her pelvis was out of alignment. I adjusted her pelvis and worked on her trigger points (trigger points are discussed in Chapter 7). When Lydia got up, the pain in her leg was gone, and she was able to bend over without pain, but her pelvic floor was still in a guarding state (increased tone), creating muscle chaos. What I mean by 'chaos' is, the muscles fire at random, often working against each other, rather than with each other. Some of them overworking, some underperforming. All, out of balance. Without addressing the pelvic floor dysfunction, the pain would come back. I showed her breathing exercises to do at home to relax her pelvic floor.

I instructed her to go home, lie on an ice pack, and do the breathing exercises up to three times a day, to continue relaxing the pelvic muscles. When she came back to my office three days later, the pain was 90% gone. She then shared with me that she has had bloating in her stomach for many years, but it had disappeared. This confirmed she suffered from CPP for long before the lift of the pot. I adjusted her again, worked on the trigger points, and showed her a few more home exercises. She continues to progress, with decreased pain, and increased function.

Chapter 2

Dr. P's Philosophy

I have been in the health field for 30 years, even so, experiencing chronic pelvic pain challenged what I thought about health and wellness, and how I treated dis-ease. My own struggle with CPP was a blessing in disguise. Being brought to a state of hopelessness around my own health and wellbeing, built a fire in me to find answers.

Your body heals from the inside out. So true healing comes from addressing our needs from the inside out. The first step is to decrease pain levels and inflammation. This gives you more relief, and the motivation to heal. It is very difficult to heal when you're in chronic pain, and a hopeless state of mind. So, the faster you can decrease pain, the more motivated you are going to be to do this program! Once the pain levels start to decrease, then we must look at diet. Specifically, at foods that cause inflammation in the body. Our major digestive organs, the intestines, sit in our pelvis. When we eat inflammatory foods, such as fried foods, this creates inflammation of the gut, which, in turn, irritates the pelvic floor, causing muscle chaos and pain.

Next, we get in touch with the muscles that support the pelvic floor. There are four key muscles in your core. The weakest of them is the pelvic floor. Balancing all muscles supports the pelvic floor. Once you gain an awareness of the pelvic floor, and other core muscles, then we can start working on *redeveloping* those muscles. If you have old patterns of chronic pain, balancing the muscles will develop healthy new patterns. Once your core is balanced and functioning together, then the strengthening comes in. If the strengthening is done too early, with a weak pelvic floor, then you will have continuous flare-ups. The base needs to be strengthened before you can start working on the power muscles. The program starts from the inside and works its way out to the larger muscles.

Introducing Dr. P's System

There could be any number of reasons why you may be experiencing pelvic pain. Even if your doctor has accurately diagnosed and successfully treated the cause, you are often left with chronic pain. Why is this?

Why your pain remains is complex, and not readily apparent. **Dr. P's System** was designed to take these complexities into consideration. Most people believe CPP is an issue of muscle weakness, or perhaps a result of not stretching enough. This, however, is dangerous assumption. If you strengthen or stretch before your body is ready, you will exacerbate any pelvic pain. You must be patient with the progress. Avoid exacerbating the problem, take it slowly, follow my program, and it will keep you on a steady path of healing.

Pelvic pain is often accompanied by a variety of new issues and symptoms. Doctors (not many) will see them as related, others will treat them as completely different conditions. As seen with Marianne and Lydia's stories, both had issues other than pelvic pain. (Marianne had numbness and tingling in her legs, Lydia had low back and leg pain.) Both were diagnosed with herniated discs. The herniated disc became the focus. However, both women were suffering from pelvic floor dysfunction, trigger points, and postural imbalances as well. Once these areas were addressed and corrected, the pain left, and function returned. Their MRI results showed both women had herniated discs. However, once their doctors diagnosed them with disc injuries, they stopped examining further. Both women were left in pain and feeling desperate.

What this system does is utilize the natural, innate, healing forces which start from the inside. We begin addressing and rehabilitating the innermost core muscle unit, then trigger points and pain patterns, then (and only then) can we strengthen the bigger muscles. You are left with stability, and muscles functioning in balance.

I have firsthand experience of the desperation that comes from going to doctors and practitioners and finding only temporary relief. The frustration that comes when nothing is changing, and you are worried you will always have limitations and pain. Let me assure you, you can get better! Maybe not 100%, but better. I would have been happy with even a 10% improvement. I was able to achieve 90% or more improvement - well beyond my expectations! The same results are possible for you too. There are many factors involved; length of time you had it; original cause; and so on. However, no matter where you are on the scale, you can improve. You can move towards muscle harmonization and optimum function.

About Dr. Pineda

I began my career in the health field in 1989, as a certified massage therapist. I had my own private practice, as well as positions in a physical therapy office, and several chiropractic offices. While practicing massage, I continued my education, eventually achieving my Doctor of Chiropractic in 2000.

My lifestyle has always been very active. Rollerblading, weight lifting, hiking, biking, traveling…. whatever I wanted to physically do, until a couple of years ago. My history includes endometriosis, which required surgery some years back. The endometriosis showed up with a fast growing, chocolate tumor. It grew from the size of a walnut to a small watermelon in three weeks. Almost overnight, I got severe inflammation in my lower abdomen. I had surgery which removed the tumor as well as an ovary. I was told they got as much of the endometriosis as possible, but there was always a chance it could come back. I did, however, continue to have inflammation in the lower abdomen. Certain foods would inflame my lower abdomen to where it would stick out as if I was carrying a small child! Very uncomfortable to say the least. An anti-inflammatory diet helped rid me of this bloating and pain. I went back to being physically active and adjusting patients again with few limitations.

I had never experienced chronic pain. I have had pain in the past, usually sports injuries which were managed by chiropractic care and exercise. That was until a couple of years ago. I started feeling pain in my hip. I thought this may be from a fall I had on my road bike a couple of years previously. Getting chiropractic adjustments would always stop the pain and free up any pelvic misalignments. The pelvic muscles would relax immediately, and the pain would go away. I felt better after adjustments and that was the end of it, so I thought.

I really didn't take the pain very seriously, since I was still able to do all the physical activities I was used to, as well as continue to physically adjust patients. But the pain always returned. This yo-yo of pain and temporary relief happened more frequently, and the level of pain increased each time. My pelvis stopped stabilizing with my usual maintenance regimen of chiropractic, massage and exercise. Then, the limitations came.

I had constant, severe pain in my low back and buttocks, to the point where any activity resulted in a flare-up. I thought my career as a chiropractor was coming to an end (as adjusting was causing a flare-up). My relationship was suffering because I was no longer able to do the activities my spouse and I liked to do together. I was desperate for a solution, and so I turned to the medical profession for special tests. My x-rays at this point were negative for any pathologies.

After a year of worsening pelvic pain, I sought help from my general practitioner. I got a pelvic MRI as well as a lumbar MRI. Both results were negative. The shocking part was that I was disappointed the MRI's were negative. I wanted so desperately to see a reason for my pain. Then I went to see my Ob-Gyn. The first OB, the surgeon who removed the endometriosis, thought it could be the endometriosis creating adhesions, which is quite common. I was in complete agreement. The pain in my pelvis was in a similar position to where I had the endometriosis removed. I was in perimenopause, so my hormones were going wild, and the OB explanation sounded feasible. They prescribed Luprin (this removes all the estrogen from your body), hoping that getting all the remaining estrogen out of my body would stop the inflammation and the pelvic pain. I welcomed this idea and had the injection of Luprin immediately. Three shots later, I did get some relief, but on a scale of 1-10, probably 1-2 in relief. Now I was in full blown menopause, with pelvic and hip pain. The endometriosis may have been the cause of this, I will never know. But what happened is that it progressed to a bigger issue. What I had hoped would be the answer just brought minimal temporary relief (the pain came back), and a whole host of new issues to deal with (hot flashes, night sweats and so on).

I then saw another OB to discuss my options. She specialized in hysterectomy surgery. We discussed options and decided to try physical therapy first with a pelvic specialist. This took three months for an appointment.

The pain started to migrate to other areas. My butt was on fire from just sitting and bending. My sacroiliac joint - that joint where your sacrum (triangular shaped bone at the base of your spine) meets with your pelvis- was constantly inflamed, and painful. My legs would throb, and I had numbness going down my leg. My low back was on fire much of the time. The pain was at a level where I was almost unable to practice as a chiropractor any longer. Trying to exercise was becoming impossible. Each time I would do an activity like hiking or biking, I would pay dearly for at least a week, with a severe flare-up. I was frustrated and feeling more than a little hopeless.

The Physical Therapist (PT) was amazing. She gave me some information that validated I was not crazy, and I started to hope I could get better. She gave me exercises which were extremely helpful, and I felt a little temporary relief. But again, the pain returned. I was still in the cycle of pain - increasing, decreasing, moderate to severe, at any given time.

Then I tried cupping which also gave me some relief. This is a form of therapy where cups are applied to the skin. This creates suction, pulling the skin and tissue up into the cup, like a reverse massage. Everything seemed to give me some relief, but nothing lasted, and I kept searching.

I came to the realization the two specialists I was seeing for treatment were not going to be able to help me when they trivialized my situation and minimized the seriousness of my deteriorating physical condition. They each told me, in almost identical words, "if this is as bad as it gets then you're going to be okay". Meaning, I wasn't going to die, so I needed to learn to live with it. This was a wakeup call for me. I knew I needed to find a solution myself. To hear I was just going to have to live with it was unacceptable to me. I had been suffering from severe pelvic, low back, and leg pain for over a year. As I began seeking my own answers, I remembered their words and used them as my motivation, the driving force, behind my search. I did find answers, and this led me to develop the *Pelvic Pain Program*. I realized I needed to be more proactive if I was going to find answers. All the activities that bring me joy exacerbated my pain levels. I have been active my entire life, if I wanted to continue to enjoy traveling, hiking, biking, and gardening, I needed to find a solution to my pain.

I was unable to accept "this is as good as it gets". Not with my background as a chiropractor, and not with my health philosophy either. As a doctor, I have always tried to help people reach their optimal level, so they can get back to the things that feed their soul. Whatever that is for them. For me it is traveling the world, which means flights sitting for long periods of time, and gardening, which is bending and lifting.

I do believe the practitioners I saw had the best of intentions. Perhaps it was how I presented, with a brave face, masking my pain and how desperate pain I was. What they told me built a fire inside me and motivated me to seek answers. That level of pain and discomfort has never been acceptable when I work with my patients, so it was not acceptable for my own health and wellbeing. I truly believe we can always improve our current condition. Maybe not resolve the issues entirely, but definitely improve. This led me to search for answers to deal with the symptoms, perhaps get to the cause, and most importantly, to live the active lifestyle I was accustomed to.

What I realized is, the cause is only part of the complexity of CPP. Yes, you should get a proper diagnosis, to see if medical intervention can stop or cure the cause. With that said, the symptoms (the pain), becomes chronic, and creates muscle chaos. Your body is either in a degenerating, or a regenerating, state. My philosophy has always been to stop the body from degenerating, and to move it into a healing state. I could not stop the degeneration that was happening in my own body. I went to five different specialists. All gave me some relief. However, the pain continued to increase, which led to a serious decrease in quality of life. To say it bluntly, I was miserable.

I was to find one more practitioner. This last practitioner (a chiropractor and nurse) had another piece of the puzzle, dry needling on the severe trigger points and specific pelvic adjustments. Trigger points are nodules in the muscle that refer pain. This gave me tremendous relief from the pain. I was then able to rehabilitate the weakened core to stabilize my pelvis and to rebalance my muscles, so my body could handle physical activity again. And the best news, I canceled the hysterectomy. The OB surgeon, PT, and the DC/RN were all very happy about this. But not nearly as happy as I was.

What I discovered, was a way to move from muscle chaos, to muscle harmonization. And I want to share it with you. My hope for you is that your pain diminishes to a level where you can function and be able to do those things in life that feed your soul. Whatever that is for you, perhaps sitting through a movie comfortably, picking up your child, swimming, biking or traveling. All those activities that give you joy.

All the practitioners I saw did their best and all gave me some temporary relief. They all wanted to help, listened to my needs, and prescribed what they do best. I am grateful to them all.

What I came to realize through all my research of CPP, is that all of the approaches are important, but that each pelvic pain sufferer is different in their cause and symptoms. Each practitioner I saw was a piece of the puzzle, but not the whole solution. Without a new approach, relief from the pain was only temporary. I didn't realize how complex the issue was with pelvic pain. I have seen many patients come to my office after their treatments have failed. Not due to the treatments being ineffective, but because only a piece of the issue was being addressed. Like Lidia with leg pain (assumed to be from a herniated disc), or Marianne who was in so much pain, pain management became the only option.

This program will give you more information than you asked for. My belief is the more you have, the better for you will be able to identify the different issues you have and get to the solution. From pain and muscle chaos to muscle harmonization, take your power back!

Chapter 3

Dr. P's Pelvic Pain Program (P4)

Whether the cause of your pelvic pain is from endometriosis like me, a physical trauma, childbirth, or something else, it doesn't matter. The pelvic pain program is designed to give you relief from the symptoms, no matter the root cause of your CPP.

The most important stabilizing sensorimotor chain (having or involving both sensory and motor functions or pathways) is the pelvic chain. You can think of this as the core unit. This system is driven from your central nervous system (your brain through your nerves) and it should be automatic. When there is a disruption in this chain, you will experience muscle chaos. The pelvic chain is the key to stability for the rest of your body; each muscle is linked intimately through the sensorimotor system. When you have pelvic dysfunction, there will be other issues to follow. You may experience strains, low back pain, knee pain, hip pain, urinary issues, and the list goes on.

Knowing the body heals from the inside out, we start from the innermost core unit muscles, and work our way out.

The pelvic floor muscles form the base of the core unit. The core unit muscles are the most important muscles, because they are your stabilizers. If there is one muscle in this group that weakens or tightens, the entire core unit will become unstable, which can trigger what I refer to as, the pelvic pain cycle. There are some muscles working too much, while others too little, often leading to increased pelvic floor tone.

The pelvic floor is controlled by the brain. The floor should contract and release automatically, without you thinking about it. Like when you cough or sneeze, the floor will contract milliseconds before, preventing the bladder from leaking. You want your pelvic floor to work automatically like this! When there is dysfunction in the floor, this automatic contraction is interrupted, often leading to bladder issues. Sometimes you don't have such noticeable symptoms, but you still have dysfunction in the pelvic floor (when this is happening, you may have no idea, until you feel pain).

The pelvic floor muscles also play an important role in supporting the pelvic organs, bladder and bowel control, and sexual function, in both men and women. When these muscles are imbalanced, you may also experience issues in these areas.

If pelvic pain and dysfunction is not addressed timely, it creates an even bigger issue. The pain continues to grow, causing trigger points. Then other muscles begin to compensate for this weakness, and the pain and dysfunction spreads to other areas of your body, as more muscles become involved. What may have started with a pelvic floor issue, now becomes an issue with your legs, your low back, and perhaps your posture. You might get sciatica, numbness or tingling in your legs, and the list goes on.

These are some common signs and symptoms you have a problem with your pelvic floor.

- Pain in the pelvic area
- Pain during sexual intercourse

- Loss of bladder control during sexual intercourse
- A prolapse
- Accidentally leaking urine when you exercise, laugh, cough or sneeze
- Needing to get to the toilet in a hurry or not making it there in time
- Finding it difficult empty your bladder or bowel
- The need to frequently go to the toilet
- Pain in your buttocks
- Pain in your legs
- Abdominal bloating
- Low back pain

When someone has pelvic floor dysfunction, the pain levels can be excruciating doing the simplest activities, such as gardening, picking up your children, or washing the dishes. When there is pelvic dysfunction, pain happens more often, and to greater levels, the longer you have it. This pain can send you running to many different specialists. Like the story of Lydia, her pelvic pain dysfunction sent her to the ER, where she was diagnosed as having a herniated disc causing sciatica. That diagnosis may have been accurate for the symptoms she was having, but the root cause was a pelvic floor weakness. The muscle relaxers and pain medication given to her certainly helped in that moment, but two days later she was back to the same place again. The pain, and the effects, would not go away unless we worked on the core issue.

This program will work for you if you are seeing a PT, chiropractor, acupuncturist, massage therapist, OBGYN, or any other specialist. This program will complement the treatment that you are already receiving, making it more effective.

Chapter 4

Restore the Floor
Beginning Pain Relief

PHASE 1: Start on the Path to Taking Back Your Life

Pelvic Floor Anatomy

Your pelvic muscle is shaped like a hammock, attached between the tailbone at the back, and the pubic bone in the front. When the pelvic floor is relaxed, it is like a relaxed hammock. When the pelvic floor is contracted, it is shortened.

Often with pelvic pain dysfunction, there is spasm in the pelvic floor, and it is unable to naturally relax. These exercises will enable you to begin to identify your pelvic floor muscles, and learn to contract, and release, them. You will also be able to identify which other muscles are compensating and begin to release them.

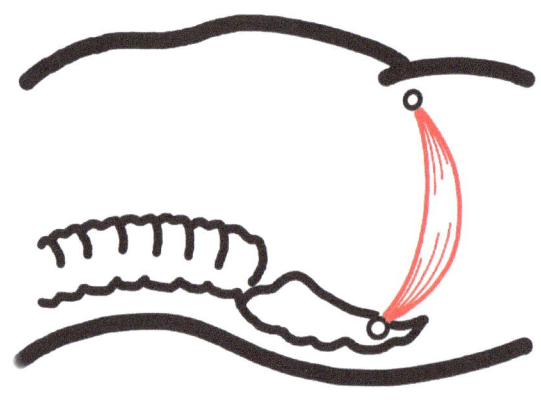
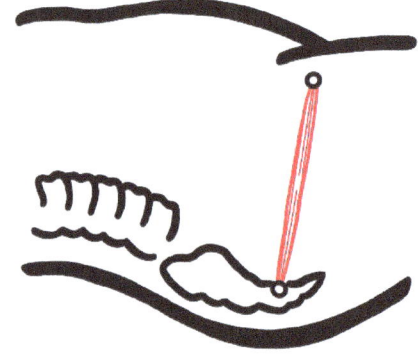

Pelvic Floor Relaxed   Pelvic Floor Contracted

Breathing Exercises

Breathing exercises are the foundation of these exercises. Master these first, before progressing. These breathing exercises are great to do in the morning before your day gets started, and then in the evening before you go to bed. The more you do them, the more you will begin to identify guarding patterns. For example, you may notice you contract your buttock muscles when you brush your teeth or wash the dishes. You can take a deep breath, and with the exhale relax those muscles. You may also notice your pelvic floor in the guarded state during various activities. Again, take a deep breath and relax those muscles with the exhale. Think of it as retraining your body how to relax.

Through these breathing exercises you will achieve the following:

1. Start rehabilitation efforts on the Inner Core

2. Begin to relax the pelvic floor muscles

3. Bring awareness of muscles that are over firing

4. Relax, and re-educate, muscles that have been engaged in compensating postural patterns

Diaphragmatic Breathing

Reps: 10   Daily: 2x

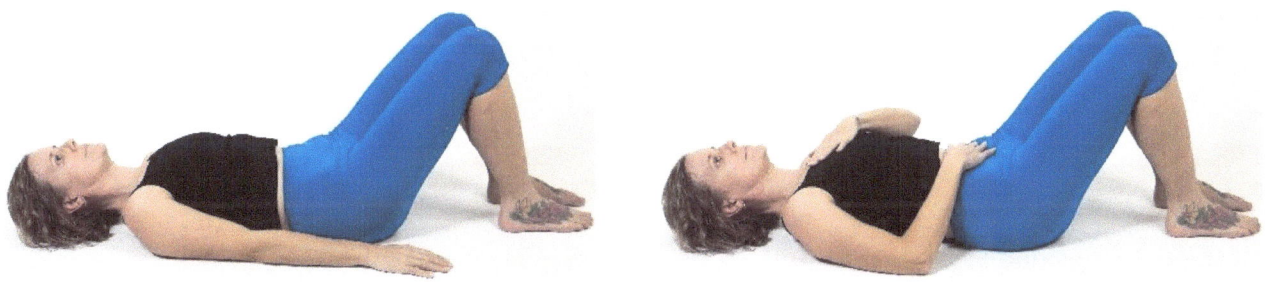

Position: Lay on your back with your knees bent, and your feet flat on the floor.

Movement: Inhale deeply into your belly only (not your chest). Focus on expanding your belly like a basketball. Exhale slowly, releasing all the air, drawing in your belly as if you are pulling your belly button toward the floor. Repeat.

Focus: Once you can inhale into your belly without engaging (filling) your chest; *focus on relaxing the muscles that you would use to hold urine and the muscles you would use to hold gas*. With the exhale, focus, and let those muscles relax. Once you can do this, keep those muscles relaxed with the inhale, as well as the exhale.

TIP: To insure only belly breathing - put one hand on your chest, the other on your belly. Focus on only the belly rising. This may take some effort. When you have pelvic pain, often the body responds with shallow breathing, only in the chest. This breathing will help get the diaphragm back to working correctly.

Note - You may feel pain in the front of your hips (hip flexors). This means these muscles have been compensating. Slide your feet further away from your butt, continue to breathe deeply. The hip flexors will begin to release. If they do not, and you feel a cramping in them (this is guarding), stretch your legs out and put a pillow under your knees. Continue your breathing with the focus on keeping the muscles that hold urine, and gas, relaxed. The hip flexors will, in time, relax.

**Your low back should remain flat on the ground. Do not let it bow. This is a compensatory postural pattern. Keep your pelvis level, do not let it twist - this is also a compensatory postural pattern we are trying to break.

*** This is the foundation for everything to come. With pelvic floor dysfunction, your pelvic floor is working overtime in a guarded state (clenching). These exercises help you begin to move in the direction of muscle harmonization.

Piriformis Stretch

Reps: 4   Hold: 30 seconds   Daily 3x

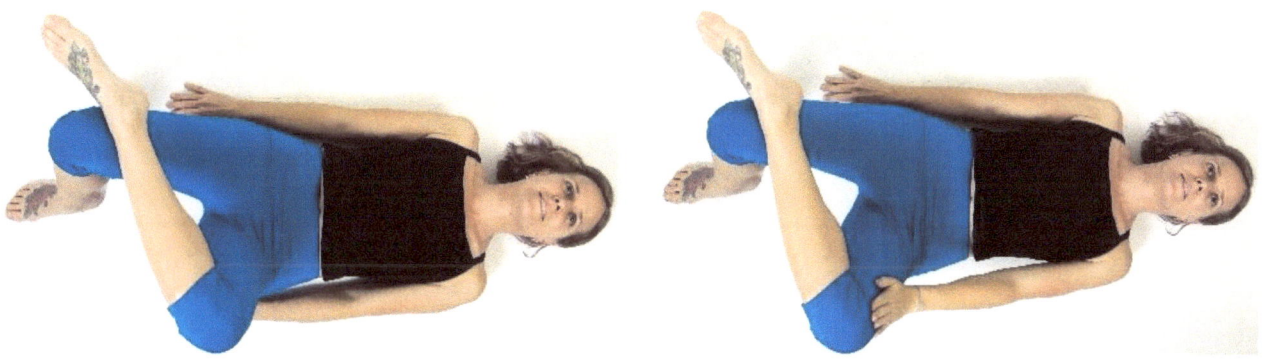

Position: Lay on your back, with both legs bent, and your feet flat on the ground.

Movement: Lift one leg and place the ankle on your opposite knee, then apply a gentle, steady pressure to your bent knee with your hand. You should not try and push the knee down. The knee will go down, most noticeably with the exhale, as the muscles in your buttocks releases.

**Your low back should remain flat on the ground. Do not let it bow. Keep your pelvis level.

Adductor Stretch

Reps: 4 Hold: 30 seconds Daily 3x

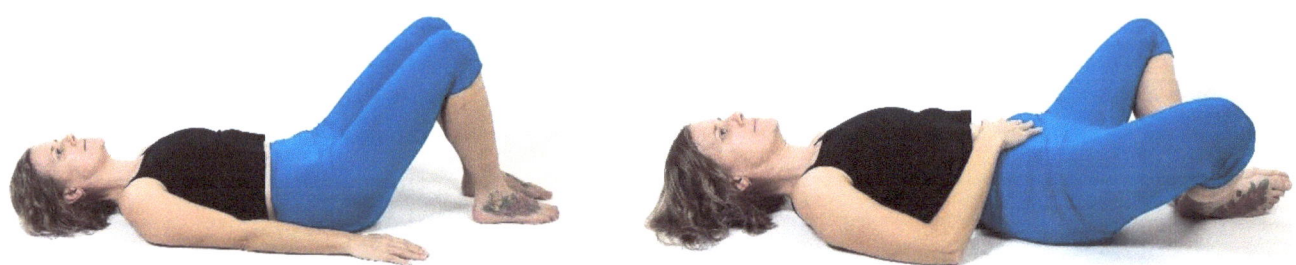

Position: Lay on your back with your knees bent, and feet on the floor. Put your feet together, sole to sole.

Movement: Let both knees slowly fall open to either side until you feel a stretch on the inside of your leg. Begin deep breathing into your belly. You will feel the muscles in your inner thighs release with the exhale.

** If these muscles are in a severe guarded state - this will be very difficult. Put a pillow on each side under your knees with the stretch. This will assist your brain/body in releasing the guarded state of the muscles, in time with your breathing

****Your low back should remain flat on the ground. Do not let it bow. Keep your pelvis level.

Pelvic Floor – Activate the Pelvic Floor Muscles

Reps: 6-10 Hold: 3 seconds Daily 2x

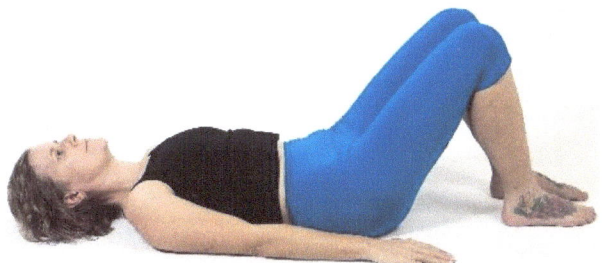

Position: Lay on your back, with your legs bent, and feet resting on the ground.

Movement: Inhale. Gently contract your lower abs and pelvic floor muscles *lightly,* and then relax with the exhale. These are the same muscles you tighten if you have to urinate but need to control your bladder - these are the pelvic floor muscles. For women, if you're comfortable using a tampon, insert one. Then using your pelvic floor and vaginal muscles, gently grip the tampon from the inside. This is the beginning of isolating the front of your pelvic floor to gain control. If you are uncomfortable with a tampon, visualize tightening those muscles.

*** Take deep diaphragmatic breaths, with slow exhales. Contract muscles with the inhale, release with the exhale.

Hip Flexor/Quad Stretch with Stretching Strap

Reps: 3 Hold: 30 seconds 1x

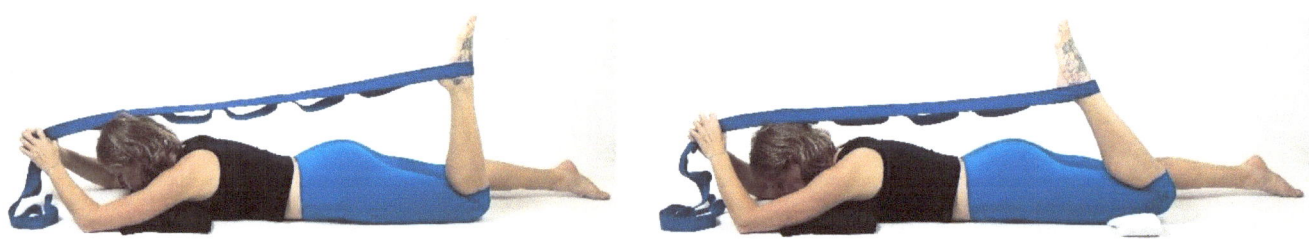

Position: Loop strap around your foot. Lie on your stomach, holding the strap. If you are very flexible, rest your knee on a rolled towel.

Movement: Gently pull the strap until you feel a stretch in your thigh and the front of your hip. Hold this position.

Contract-release technique: Push your pubic bone gently into the floor.

At the same time, gently push your knee into the floor. Relax these muscles, then pull the strap to stretch the thigh and front of the hip.

**Important: Make sure your glutes (buttocks) are relaxed. They may be in a guarded state. Keep diaphragmatic breathing, release the glutes with the exhale. This will help with any compensatory postures of your glutes.

Hip Stretch, Pelvic Floor Lengthener

Reps: 4 Hold: 15 seconds Daily 3x

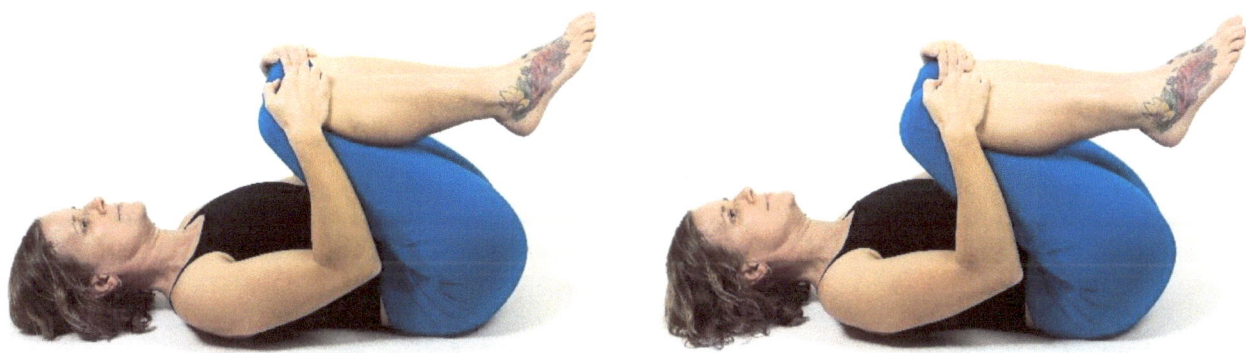

Position: Lay on your back, with your knees towards your chest. Hold your knees.

Movement: Gently pull your legs towards your chest. Breathe deep diaphragmatic breaths, focusing on the pelvic floor and buttock muscles staying relaxed.

Pelvic Alignment

Pelvic dysfunction is a multifaceted condition, requiring concurrent treatments. I believe, the most important one to be pelvic alignment. The pelvis is the source of your strength. It is your center. You use it for lifting, pushing, pulling, and getting up from a seated position. The pelvis is integral to good posture and body alignment. If your pelvis is rotated forward, the curve in your low back will flatten, and your head will thrust forward, giving you a hunched posture. Your gait will be off, and your leg will swing out, instead of forward. Misalignment of the pelvis creates a distortion and causes nerve disturbances. Whatever is at the end of those nerves will suffer dysfunction as a result. For example, some people with pelvic problems get referral pain down the side of the leg or in the top of the leg area.

Distortions in the pelvis can affect the pelvic floor, as the body tries to adapt to a constant torque or a constant pressure on the pelvis. The muscles constantly engage, or guard, and you have neuromechanical dysfunction, meaning movement is distorted. This is a natural physiological response; the body is trying to protect you from further injury. However, this is not how a normal body should function, and is a precursor to a host of other issues. This is the start of a downward spiral of degeneration, muscle sprains and strains, compensatory patterns, trigger points (I talk about trigger points in the pain relief chapter), and pelvic floor dysfunction. You may have distortions in the pelvis for years before the symptoms show up or it may be just a short time. It may have originated from a fall, from being pregnant, or the birthing process itself.

The myriad of symptoms manifested from a misaligned pelvis will often lead to a misdiagnosis of the underlying issue. Pelvic misalignment can cause groin pain, pubic pain, constipation, painful periods, poor circulation in legs and feet, pain changing positions from sitting to standing, pain lying down and pelvic floor issues! The wide variety of symptoms often leads doctors to (incorrectly) give a diagnosis that fits the particular symptom you are presenting, not understanding the root cause is a misaligned pelvis.

As a chiropractor, I specialize in this area. After a chiropractic adjustment, the pelvis starts moving and the muscles relax. They don't have to guard anymore and neuromechanical function is restored. Without a chiropractic adjustment, the pelvic muscles remain under stress, resulting in constant asymmetrical muscle contractions. The muscles become tendinous (or tighter) to stabilize the area. Chronicity sets in. Some muscles shorten, others overwork and become strained. Ligaments are affected and sprained. Trigger points emerge. Pelvic floor dysfunction develops. Any pelvic floor organs can also be affected; the reproductive organs, the urinary bladder, the colon, and the rectum.

I suggest you seek a chiropractor to join your personal wellness team. Find someone who either does x-rays, or sends you out for them, and who can read them. Radiographs are the only way to show exactly how your pelvis is misaligned. They also show other important information. Without an x-ray, you are blind. At this point in your healing, you have suffered enough, and guess work has no place. Make sure the radiographs are weight bearing (taken standing up), to show what your pelvis does with your body weight. Your pelvis may look perfect when you lay down, but as soon as you stand, it twists. The longer you have a misaligned spine coupled with inflammation, the more degeneration you will get. The pelvis joints can fuse with long term dysfunction. If at all possible you want to catch pelvic distortion before it gets to this point.

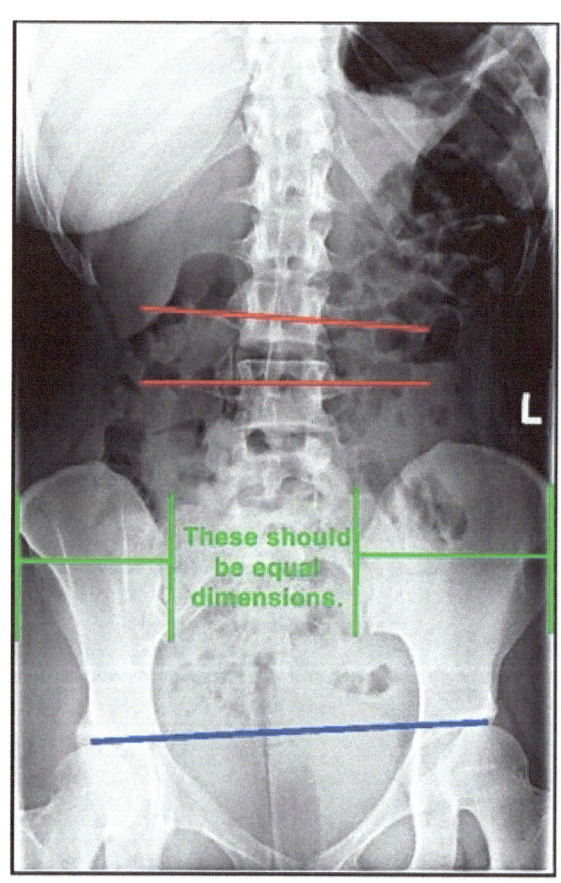

Black spots are painful gas build up in the gut.

Twisted Pelvis

Causes groin pain, constipation, painful periods, poor circulation in the legs and feet, pain changing positions from sitting to standing, pain walking.

Pelvis is not level

Creates pain and degeneration in the back, hip, knee, and/or foot from unbalanced gait. Joints wear out or injure more on one side of the body.

Chapter 5

Preventing Flare-Ups

PHASE 2 – Control the Controllable

Identify your triggers to prevent constant flare-ups

Triggers are the activities that cause flare-ups in your condition (increased pain and dysfunction). I will give you a couple of examples of mine.

I have a great road bicycle and love to ride. I thought the pain would increase from the position you have to be in to ride a road bike, but the more I learned, it is definitely from sitting on the hard seat. When riding, you are sitting on your pelvic floor. If there is increased spasming (tone), it will only get worse! Hiking was another favorite activity of mine, and sure enough, hiking uphill caused an increase in my pain. My pelvis was not level, and the muscles did not work as they should. I would feel my abdominal muscles twitch uncontrollably when I rested. My hamstrings and groin muscle would fire painfully. Then the pain would last for weeks.

There are a couple of problems with a flare-up. One, it lasts for a good couple of weeks, two, it involves more muscles, and increases poor posture patterns, which, you guessed it, increases pain levels.

Here is a list of possible physical triggers to look out for, and solutions to help you prevent a flare-up:

- Prolonged sitting
    - Get a sit stand station if you have to sit at work. At home, get up periodically. Avoid long driving trips. If you have to, stop periodically to relieve the pressure on your pelvic floor.
- Walking uphill
    - If you can avoid this, do. You will be able to walk uphill once you get a properly functioning pelvis that is level and your muscles are working in balance.
- Bending over
    - Use the SI Joint Brace *
- Squatting
    - Use the SI Joint brace to support your pelvis
- Vacuuming
    - Use the SI Joint brace to support your pelvis
- Doing dishes
    - Use the SI Joint brace to support your pelvis

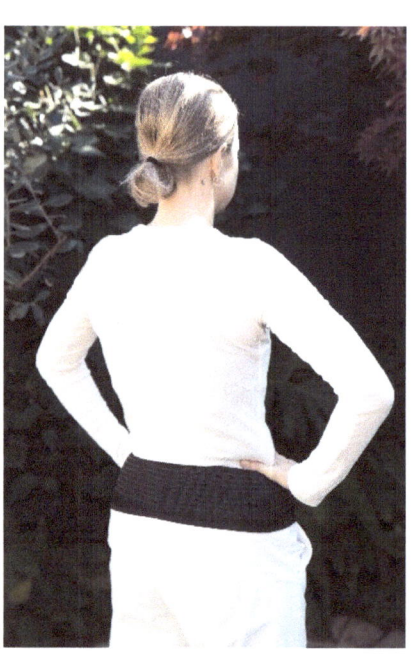

*Note: You can test yourself to see if a SI Joint Brace will help you. Ask a friend or loved one (using light but firm pressure) to grip each hip and gently squeeze each side of your pelvis towards your midline. If you feel relief, your pelvis is unstable. Use the belt when doing physical activities including washing dishes and vacuuming to help. When your pelvis stabilizes after the strengthening portion of the program, you can stop using it.

- Lying on your side
    - Use a side pillow between your legs

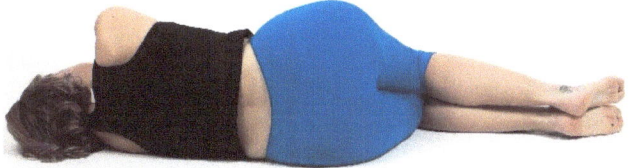 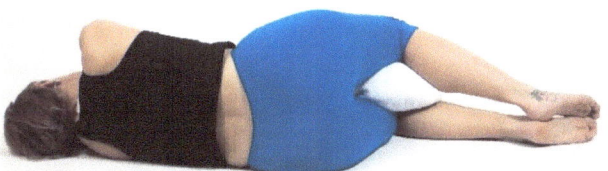

No knee pillow, pelvic muscles are stretched   With knee pillow, pelvic muscles relaxed

- Sitting with a wallet in your back pocket
    - Don't do it!
- Sitting in a minimally supportive chair ie: lawn chair
    - Again, don't do it.
- Crossing legs when sitting

Don't do it. You are stressing your pelvis, lengthening some muscles and putting unbalanced weight on your pelvis.

- Putting on socks or pants from a standing position
    - Sit and pull your socks and pants on. Otherwise, you can pull the glutes, or overload the gluteal muscles, on the weight-bearing side.
- Inflammatory foods
    - If you have IBS, endometriosis, or other inflammatory conditions; inflammatory foods exacerbate these conditions, which adds to the irritation in the pelvis

*See list of possible inflammatory foods in the next section on gut health

- Over stretching inflamed muscles

- This actually does the opposite of your goal. Over stretching an injured muscle kick starts the body's natural guarding system, increasing tone. Increased tone leads to additional trigger points and postural compensation.
- Strength training with a weak core
  - With an imbalance in your core, you become very susceptible to further injury. Work on balancing your core first, following my exercises, then move on to strength training.

Chapter 6

Gut Health

What you eat plays a critical role in your health. How many times have you heard this before? Unfortunately, even though we all should know this, it is often overlooked. Inflammation of the gut can trigger a flare-up just as much as physical activity can. Gut health cannot be ignored.

People with pelvic floor issues often have gut issues. Some of the more common symptoms associated with gut problems are bloating, gas, constipation, diarrhea, cramping and abdominal pain. An inflamed gut sitting in the pelvis, irritating the pelvic floor, causes increased tone (spasms). This in turn, can cause spasm and irritation to the structures and organs that sit in the pelvic region. These structures and organs include, loops of the small intestine, colon, rectum, anal canal, bladder, lower part of the urethra, and the reproductive organs. So gut health must be a part of pelvic floor rehabilitation. It starts with the food you eat.

You can improve your gut health immediately by eliminating these Top Five Foods which are major contributors to gut inflammation:

- Corn
- Soy
- Pork
- Wheat
- Dairy

Corn is a grain and extremely inflammatory. There are also other health reasons for eliminating corn from your diet. 88 percent of corn is genetically modified[6]. This enables it to be sprayed with a powerful herbicide that will destroy the weeds, while the corn will survive. Herbicides are toxic. Do what you can to avoid consuming food sprayed by herbicides and pesticides. Corn is also used to feed chickens, cows, and pigs. They ingest the herbicide, and then you ingest them! High-fructose corn syrup is hidden in a lot of foods; this is yet another way toxins are quietly getting into your system. Start reading the labels of your food.

Some of the most common corn by-product names you will find on many labels[7]:

- Corn flour, cornmeal, corn gluten, cornflakes
- Cornstarch, also listed on labels as starch or vegetable starch
- Corn oil
- Dextrins, Maltodextrins, Dextrose
- Fructose or crystalline fructose
- Hydrol, treacle
- Ethanol
- Free fatty acids
- Maize
- Zein
- Sorbitol

---

[6] (Kelly, 2012)
[7] (Pediatrics, 2018)

Soy, the second food on our list of inflammatory foods, is commonly found in tofu, soy milk, soy sauce, and many vegetarian meat substitutes. 93% of all soy is genetically modified[8]. Soy became popular in the early 2000's shortly after a study of low breast cancer rates in Japanese women was released. The study correlated the consumption of soy, miso soup, and isoflavones with breast cancer. The study found that frequent miso soup and isoflavone consumption reduced the risk of breast cancer, however, there was no evidence that soy reduced the risk of breast cancer, yet this conclusion seems to have been missed! While there may be some health benefits from fermented soy, soy found commonly in the United States is unfermented. The difference is in the processing. Unfermented soy products contain phytic acid, a type of antinutritional component that interferes with nutrient absorption and irritates the lining of the gut, becoming a big contributor to gut inflammation. Unfortunately, soy is commonly used in food production as a filler. Read food labels carefully and know what you are putting in your body.

Pork, number three on our list, is high in inflammatory Omega-6 fats. Omega-3 is anti-inflammatory, Omega-6 is inflammatory. We need Omega-6 in our diet, however the ratio of Omega-3 to Omega-6 is so out of proportion in the American diet that Omega-6's can almost be thought of as bad. (They are not, of course, when consumed in the right ratio). In the United States, pigs mostly eat grains and seed oils, which greatly increases their Omega-6 content as well as arachidonic acid. Both are highly inflammatory for your gut. In consuming pig meat, you are also ingesting what the pig ate. "You are what you eat" is a common, and true saying. Another issue is that pork is generally processed, either preserved by smoking, curing or salting, or adding

---

[8] (J Natl Cancer Inst., 2003)

potentially harmful chemicals. Think smoked ham, bacon, processed lunch meats, and sausage. You are consuming the chemicals used to process these foods.

Wheat, number four on our list, is also an inflammatory food commonly found in many items on the supermarket shelf. Unless someone has Celiac disease, consumed in whole or cracked form, (Non-GMO) grains do not necessarily cause inflammation or damage the gut. But when they are milled into flour, they become high-glycemic which converts them into sugars and protein, making them pro-inflammatory. Studies have shown wheat contributes to the manifestation of chronic inflammation and autoimmune diseases, and chronic health conditions, by increasing intestinal permeability and initiating a pro-inflammatory immune response[9]. Note that whole wheat flour and whole wheat bread is not whole or cracked form wheat!

Dairy, the last of our Top Five Inflammatory Foods, could also be a triggering food. It has been estimated that 75 percent of people will become lactose intolerant at some point in their lives[10]. Consuming dairy will result in bloating, abdominal cramps, and gas. If you have gut issues already, Irritable Bowel Syndrome, Crohn's disease, Endometriosis, or other gut conditions, dairy may trigger flare-ups of these conditions and CPP. There is no "gold standard" test available to diagnosis lactose intolerance. You can do an elimination test to see if you cannot digest dairy.

After you have eliminated the five major inflammatory foods listed above, identify and remove these popular foods that also trigger inflammation in your body.

- Processed foods (most are full of soy and corn)

---

[9] (de Punder & Pruimboom, 2013)
[10] (Mattar, de Campos Mazo, & Carrilho, 2012)

- Sugar
- Trans fats (found in fried foods)
- Refined carbs (found in white bread, white pasta, and pastries)
- Soybean oil and vegetable oil
- Processed snack foods, such as chips and crackers
- Desserts, cookies, candy, ice cream
- Excess alcohol

Instead, eat foods that are anti-inflammatory. These include:
- Beans and lentils
- Pineapple
- Blueberries, blackberries, and cherries
- Green leafy vegetables, including kale and spinach
- Broccoli and cauliflower
- Beets
- Avocado
- coconut
- Olives
- Extra virgin olive oil
- Walnuts, pistachios, pine nuts, and almonds (raw)
- Cold water fish, including salmon (not farmed – farmed fish are fed grains which are high in Omega 6) and sardines
- Turmeric and cinnamon
- Dark chocolate
- Green Tea

Avoid sugary drinks and be sure to stay hydrated with water.

In order to clear your body of all the toxic food and chemicals, you can try a 30-day clean eating plan. This will remove foods that may be causing inflammation and symptoms and give your body a chance to heal. This will help you to determine which foods cause symptoms or give you a negative reaction. This is a powerful tool so you can discover which foods directly flare-up your CPP symptoms.

Sample recipes of an anti-inflammatory diet are provided at the end of the book.

Fasting to Decrease Inflammation

Once I started feeling better and was able to perform physical activities again, I still felt sluggish. My energy was down, and I had a "foggy" brain, I attributed this to menopause. I had gained about 15 pounds. I had already changed my diet to an anti- inflammatory diet, and yet I still could not shake the sluggish feeling. I was able to exercise again, but really was not motivated! Then came the next step in gut health for me, fasting. I remembered reading research on fasting with amazing results some years back and watching a documentary on the benefits of fasting. Though the results were profound, I thought at the time, I would not be able to fast. I need to be sharp and present at work while seeing patients. I did not think I could maintain the level of patient care I wanted to provide if I was fasting.

That was then, and now I have discovered more recent research. I found a fasting program that tricks your brain into thinking you are fasting while you are on a limited calorie diet. This provides all the benefits of fasting, but you are able to sustain muscle and brain function. I was all for this and eager to try it out. I have now fasted several times, and it worked! I was finally able to boost my metabolism and clear the brain 'fog'. Most importantly, the fasting reduces inflammation, which is the biggest benefit.

One study demonstrated that a periodic 3-day cycle of a fasting reduced levels of pro-inflammatory cytokines[11]. Another study concluded intermittent fasting, and caloric restriction, extends life expectancy, and reduces inflammation and cancer risk[12]. For so long I felt like I was drifting away from wellness, and into a spiral of degeneration. Fasting arrested that trend. I have lost 14lbs and my energy is up and my mind clear. The best part is not the weight loss, but the decrease in gut inflammation.

Fasting:

- Improves energy levels
- Helps maintain healthy levels of cholesterol
- Helps maintain healthy levels of inflammation
- Lowers body fat
- Supports weight loss
- Helps maintain lean body mass
- Helps maintain healthy levels of blood glucose and blood pressure
- Reduces waist size and lowers abdominal fat

Don't try this on your own. There are very unhealthy ways to fast and there are also great programs out there. I recommend you do your own research in this area and speak to your physician to see if fasting is right for you.

---

[11] (Cell Reports, 2016)
[12] (Faris, et al., 2012)

Chapter 7

Pain Relief Naturally!

Phase 3 – Relieve Chronic Pain
Trigger Points are a BIG Deal

A 'Trigger Point' is, (a focus of hyperirritability in a tissue that, when compressed, is locally tender and, if sufficiently hypersensitive, gives rise to referred pain and tenderness)[13].

Understanding, and dealing with, trigger points is critical for pain management. When we have altered postures (compensatory postures) due to pain in the pelvis region, some muscles begin to work too hard, while other muscles not hard enough. Compensatory postures overload some muscles. When this happens, trigger points develop. Trigger points create pain. You can actually feel a trigger point if you know where it is. It feels like a little nodule. When this hypersensitive tissue becomes irritated, it refers pain to other regions of your body. When you're looking at the pictures of the different trigger points in your body, you can see that the region of pain might go over three quarters of your leg, from just one trigger point! It *feels* like you now have a leg issue, when before you just had pelvic pain. Now you feel it down your leg, and you think the problem is more than the pelvis. This is the issue with chronic pelvic pain. Once you feel the pain spreading you think that the problem is getting bigger, and that you're never going to get better.

---

[13] (Travell, MD & Simons MD, Myofascial Pain and Dysfunction. The Trigger Point Manual. The Lower Extremities., 1992)

But understanding what trigger points are, and how they can develop, stops this line of thinking. Trigger points can be dealt with, and they can be decreased. When a trigger point shrinks, the pain decreases almost immediately, and your range of motion increases. What a relief!

By learning about trigger points, you will understand, one, there is an answer and you can decrease trigger point pain, and two, the chronic pain, or the feeling that the problem is only getting bigger, will make sense to you. If we can deal with these trigger points and decrease them, then reduce the inflammation, and finally get the pelvic floor and core muscles to relax and start functioning correctly, then you will see how you will start moving in the direction of health and healing. You can move away from a life of chronic pain.

There are several different ways to deal with trigger points. It depends on how long you've had them and how bad they are. If you just started this journey with pelvic pain, you may have just a few trigger points that can be dealt with fairly easily. But if you've been dealing with this for a long time, maybe years, you probably have trigger points all over your body, and many in the lower extremities. It may take longer, and it may be more challenging, to get them dealt with, but we can do it. I'm going to go through different ways that you can address trigger points, and you'll decide what works for you. Some are very effective when you're at home and you can't get out. You can do this trigger point therapy on yourself, or if you have a practitioner available to help you relieve these trigger points, that's good too.

Mapping Trigger Points

These following images map out where trigger points are and where you may experience referred pain from the trigger points. In the following illustrations, the trigger point locations are noted as circles. The areas of primary and referred pain you may be feeling associated with the trigger point are depicted as solid and diffused patterns in the illustration. Trigger points can refer to other parts of your body, for example an abdominal trigger point can refer pain to your low back.

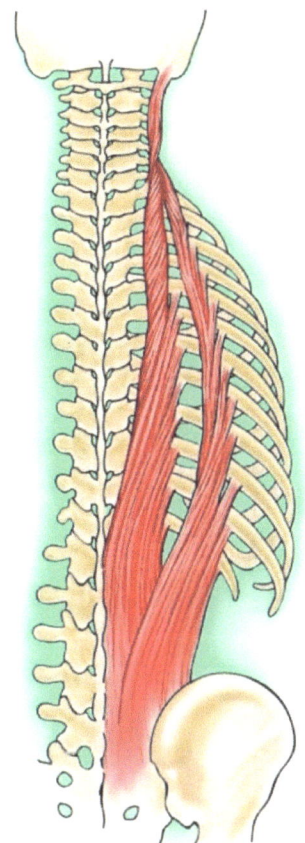

Figure 7.1

Superficial Paraspinal Muscles

An issue with your pelvis can affect other areas of your spine and body. Trigger points can develop in the superficial paraspinal muscles (Figure 7.1).

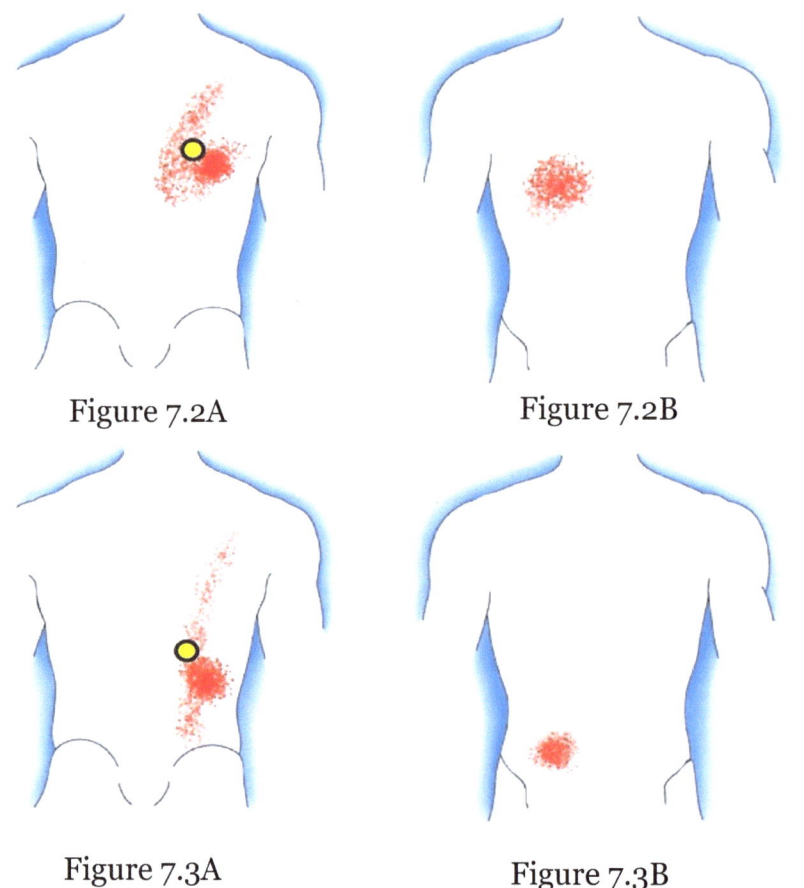

Figure 7.2A   Figure 7.2B

Figure 7.3A   Figure 7.3B

Iliocostalis Thoracis muscle trigger points refer pain into the scapular region (Figure 7.2A) and may also refer pain in the front chest (Figure 7.2B). The lower Iliocostalis Thoracis muscle trigger point (Figure 7.3A) refers pain down the low back to the top of the ilium and up to the lateral scapular region. Referred pain can also be felt in the front lower quadrant of the abdomen (Figure 7.3B).[14]

---

[14] (Travell, MD & Simons, MD, Myofascial Pain and Dysfunction. The Trigger Point Manual. The Upper Extremities., 1983)

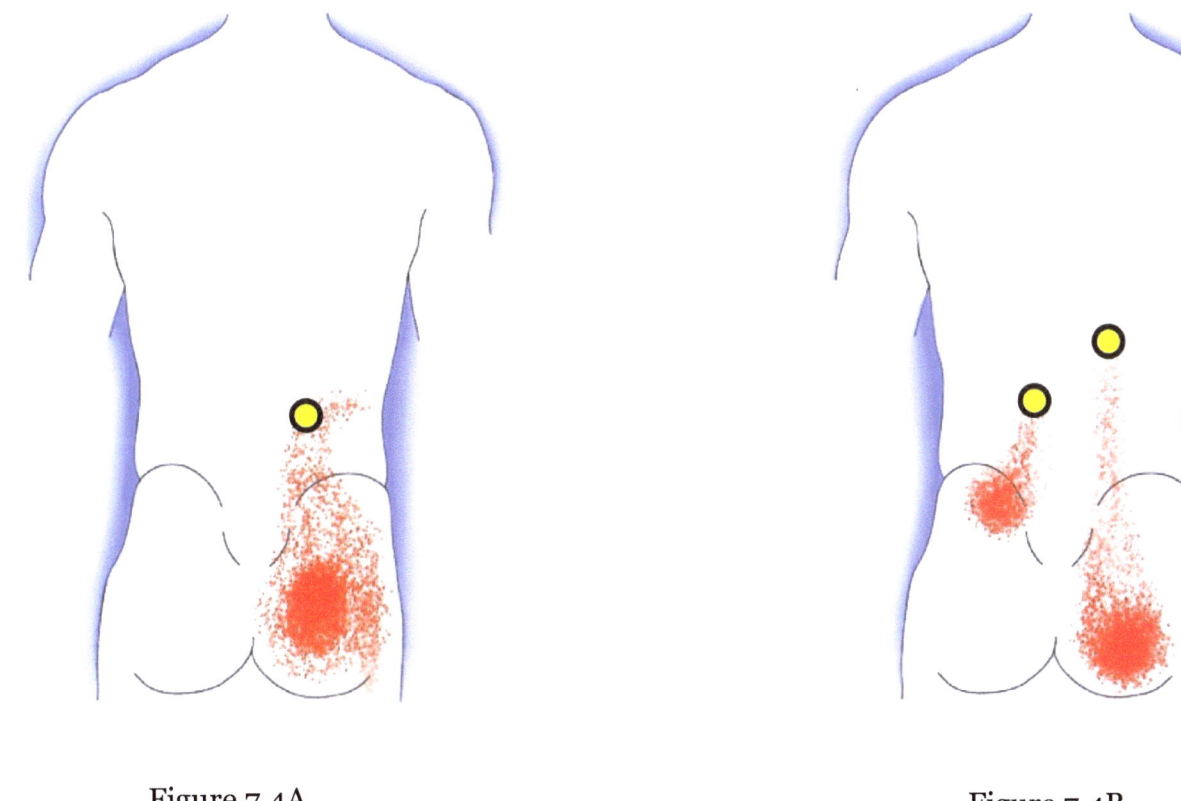

Figure 7.4A   Figure 7.4B

The Iliocostalis Lumborum muscle trigger points refer pain into your low back and buttocks (glutes) (Figure 7.4A, and Figure 7.4B) and the top of the hip (Figure 7.4A).[15]

---

[15] (Travell, MD & Simons, MD, Myofascial Pain and Dysfunction. The Trigger Point Manual. The Upper Extremities., 1983)

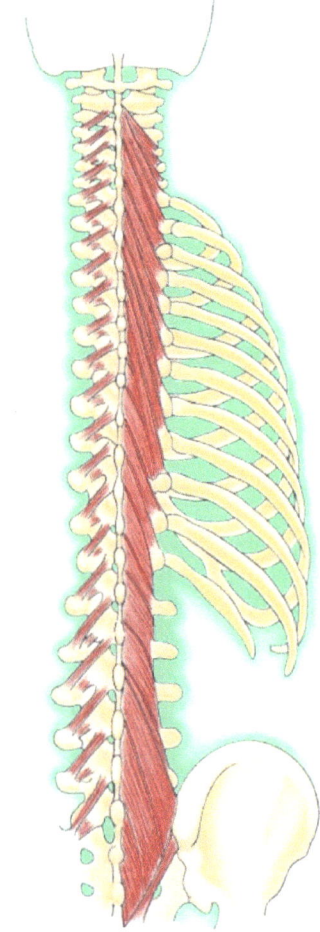

Figure 7.5

Spine Multifidi muscles (Figure 7.5). The posterior muscles of the Core Unit.

An imbalance of the core can cause the multifidi to develop trigger points, this creates an even bigger issue of pain and imbalance. The following images (Figure 7.5A, Figure 7.5B, and Figure 7.5C) show where these trigger points can develop and refer pain.

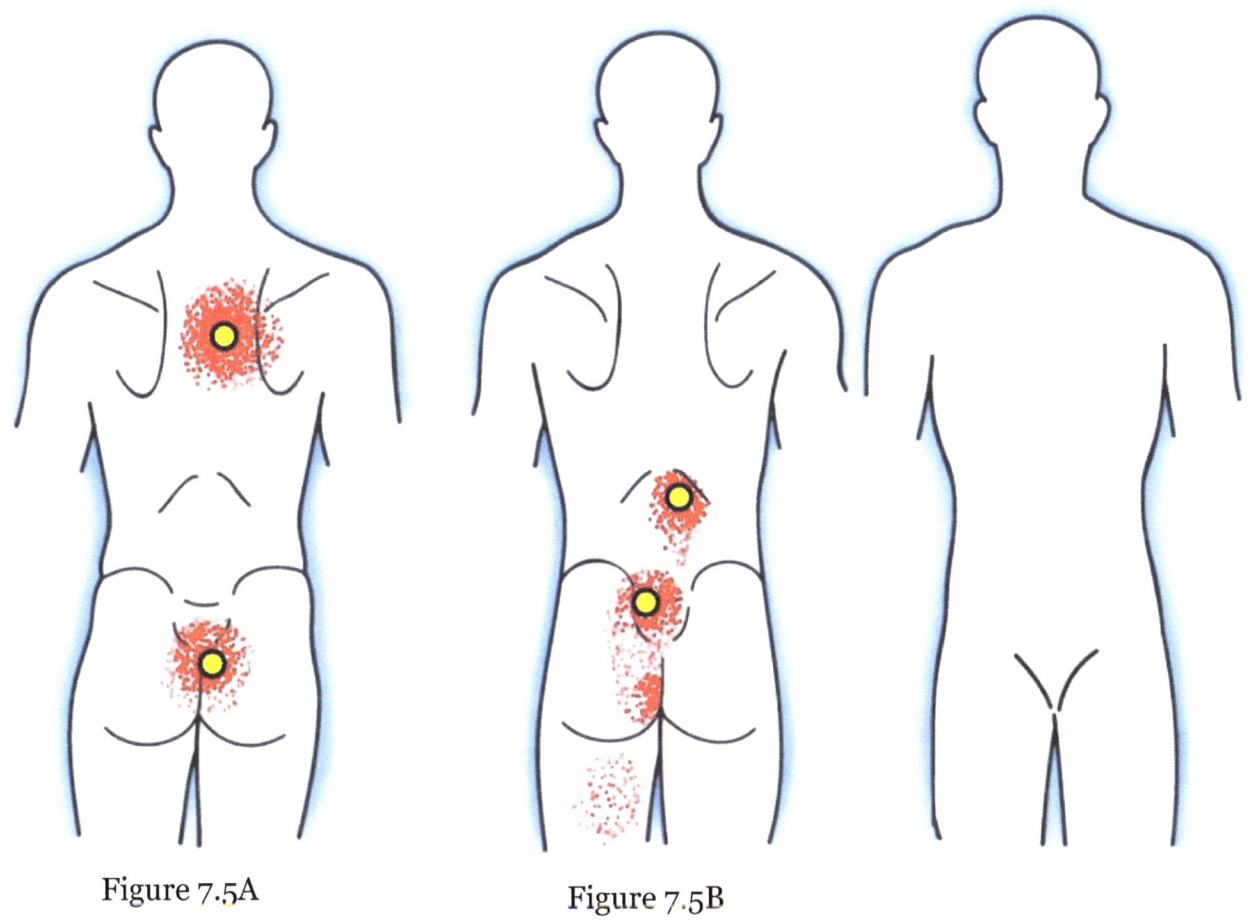

Figure 7.5A   Figure 7.5B

Multifidi muscle trigger points (Figure 7.5A, and Figure 7.5B) in the spinal muscles refer pain into the coccyx and mid back (Figure 7.5A) and low back (Figure 7.5B). Pain can refer down from the sacrum to the back of the thigh (Figure 7.5B). [16]

---

[16] (Travell, MD & Simons, MD, Myofascial Pain and Dysfunction. The Trigger Point Manual. The Upper Extremities., 1983)

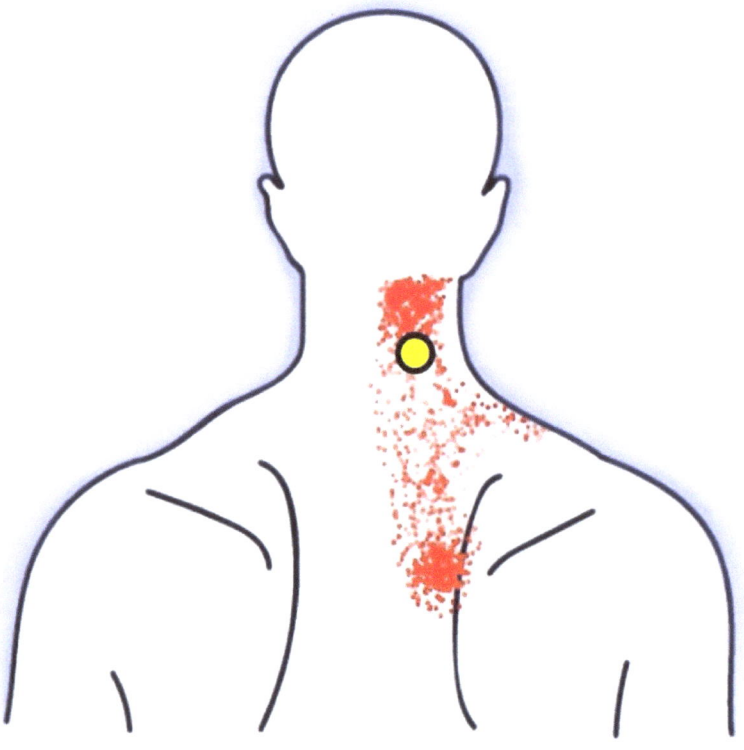

Figure 7.5C

With the multifidi muscles affected from pelvic floor dysfunction, the upper multifidi muscle trigger point in the neck (cervical spine) (Figure 7.5C) can refer pain into the neck, across the trap and down into the scapular region.[17] This can produce neck pain, headaches, neck stiffness, and so on!

---

[17] (Travell, MD & Simons, MD, Myofascial Pain and Dysfunction. The Trigger Point Manual. The Upper Extremities., 1983)

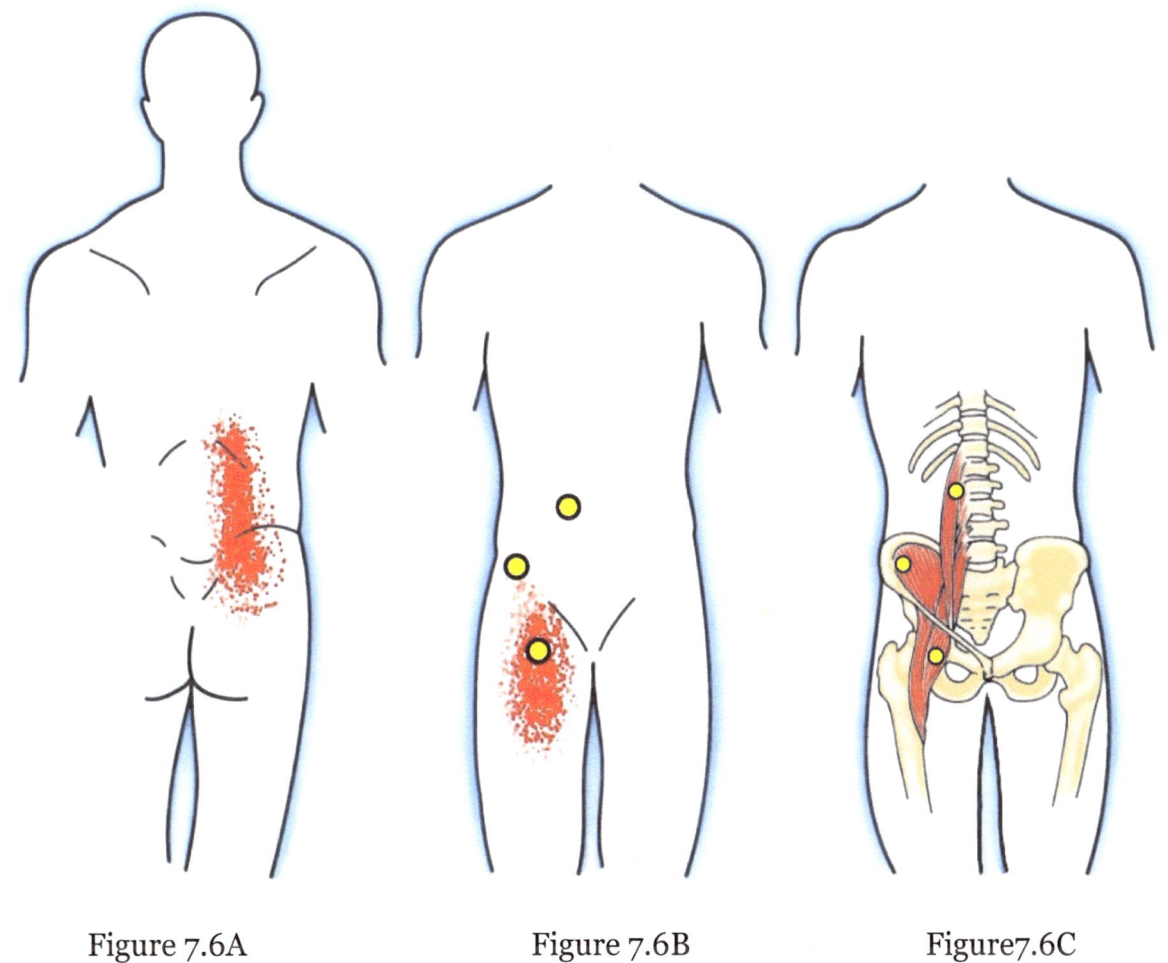

Figure 7.6A   Figure 7.6B   Figure 7.6C

Iliopsoas muscle trigger points (Figure 7.6C) refer pain into the low back along the lumbar spine, into the upper glutes (Figure 7.6A) and in the front lower abdomen to the top of leg (flexors) (Figure 7.6B).[18]

---

[18] (Travell, MD & Simons MD, Myofascial Pain and Dysfunction. The Trigger Point Manual. The Lower Extremities., 1992)

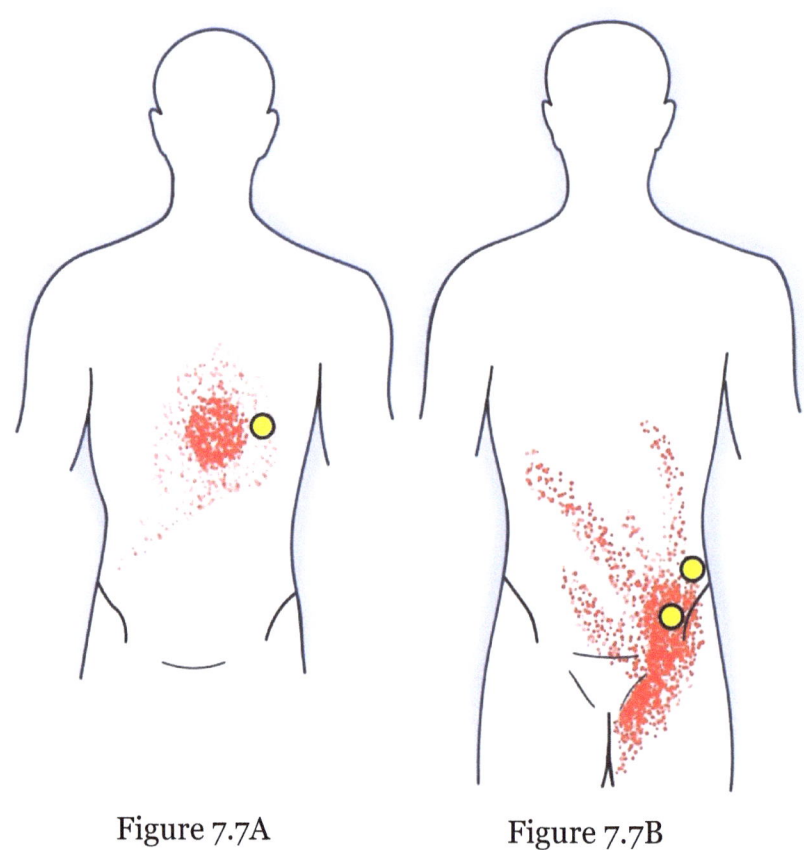

Figure 7.7A Figure 7.7B

Upper Abdominal Oblique trigger points (Figure 7.7A) can radiate pain in the upper abdomen and lower chest region, producing symptoms like those of heartburn and hiatal hernia. Lower Abdominal Oblique trigger points (Figure 7.7B) can radiate pain across the abdominal muscles and down the groin region into your genitalia.[19]

---

[19] (Travell, MD & Simons, MD, Myofascial Pain and Dysfunction. The Trigger Point Manual. The Upper Extremities., 1983)

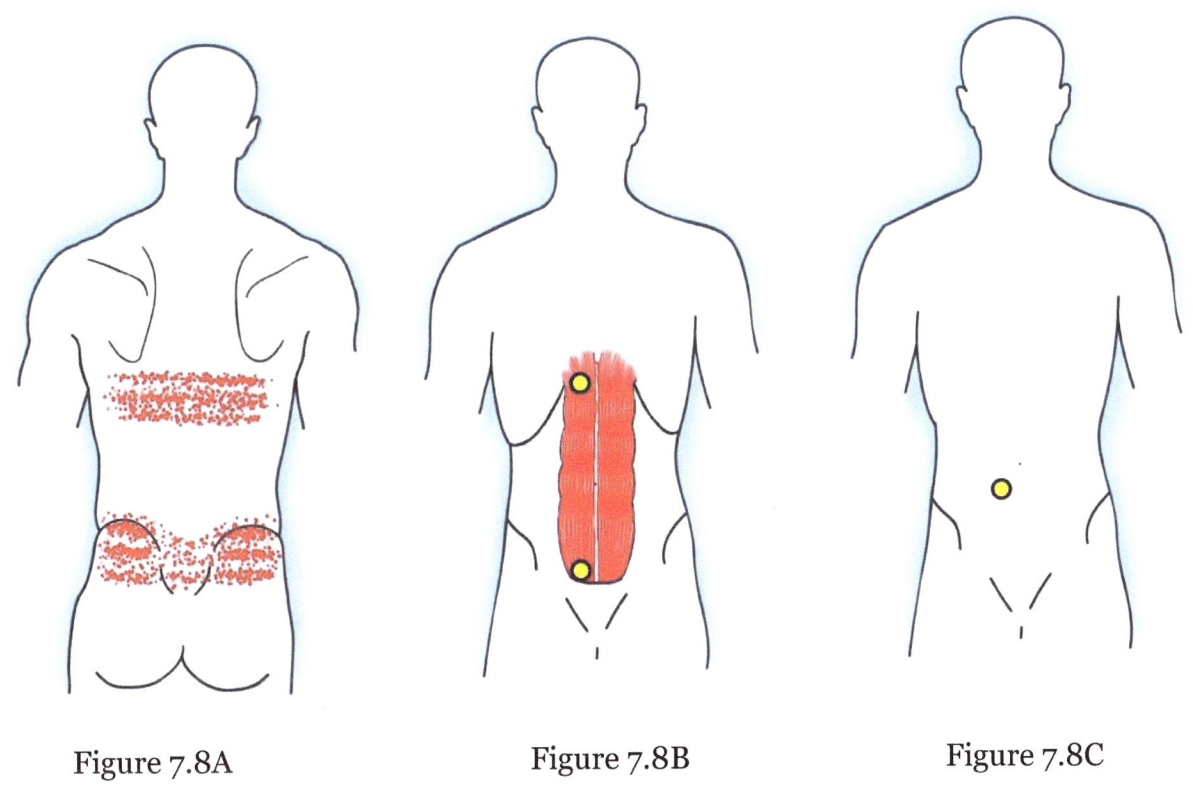

Figure 7.8A   Figure 7.8B   Figure 7.8C

Rectus Abdominis trigger points (Figure 7.8B and Figure 7.8C) can refer pain into your mid-back in a bandlike pain pattern and across the hips and sacrum (Figure 7.8A).[20]

---

[20] (Travell, MD & Simons, MD, Myofascial Pain and Dysfunction. The Trigger Point Manual. The Upper Extremities., 1983)

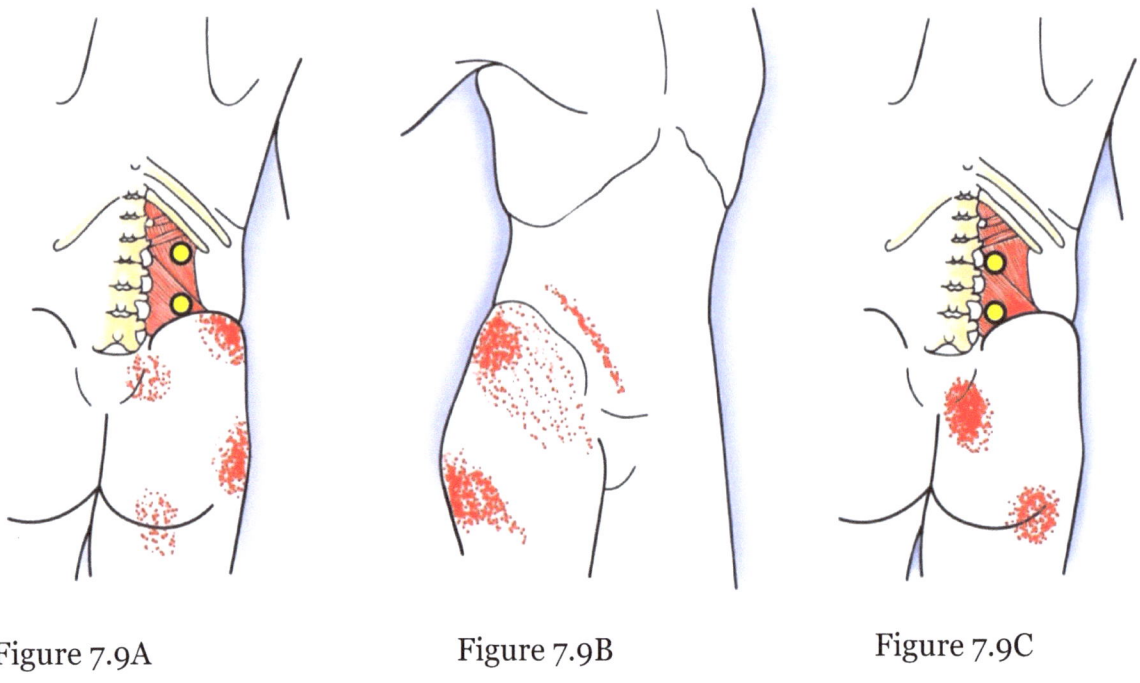

Figure 7.9A   Figure 7.9B   Figure 7.9C

Quadratus Lumborum (QL) trigger points (Figure 7.9A) refer pain along the top and side of the hip to the front to the groin region (Figure 7.9B). Trigger points also refer pain into the sacroiliac joint (Figure 7.9C). QL trigger points can create sharp, shooting pain, when moving the hips and pelvis.[21]

---

[21] (Travell, MD & Simons MD, Myofascial Pain and Dysfunction. The Trigger Point Manual. The Lower Extremities., 1992)

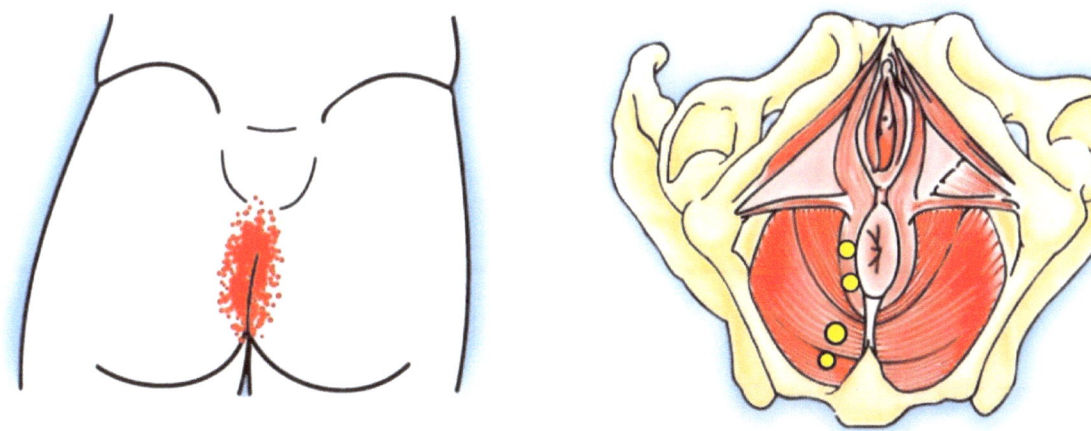

Figure 7.10A   Figure 7.10B

Pelvic Floor – Sphincter Ani, Levator Ani and Coccygeous trigger points (Figure 7.10B) refer pain to the lower coccyx and the anal region (Figure 7.10A). Trigger points in the anterior half of the pelvic floor are likely to refer pain to the genitalia.[22]

---

[22] (Travell, MD & Simons MD, Myofascial Pain and Dysfunction. The Trigger Point Manual. The Lower Extremities., 1992)

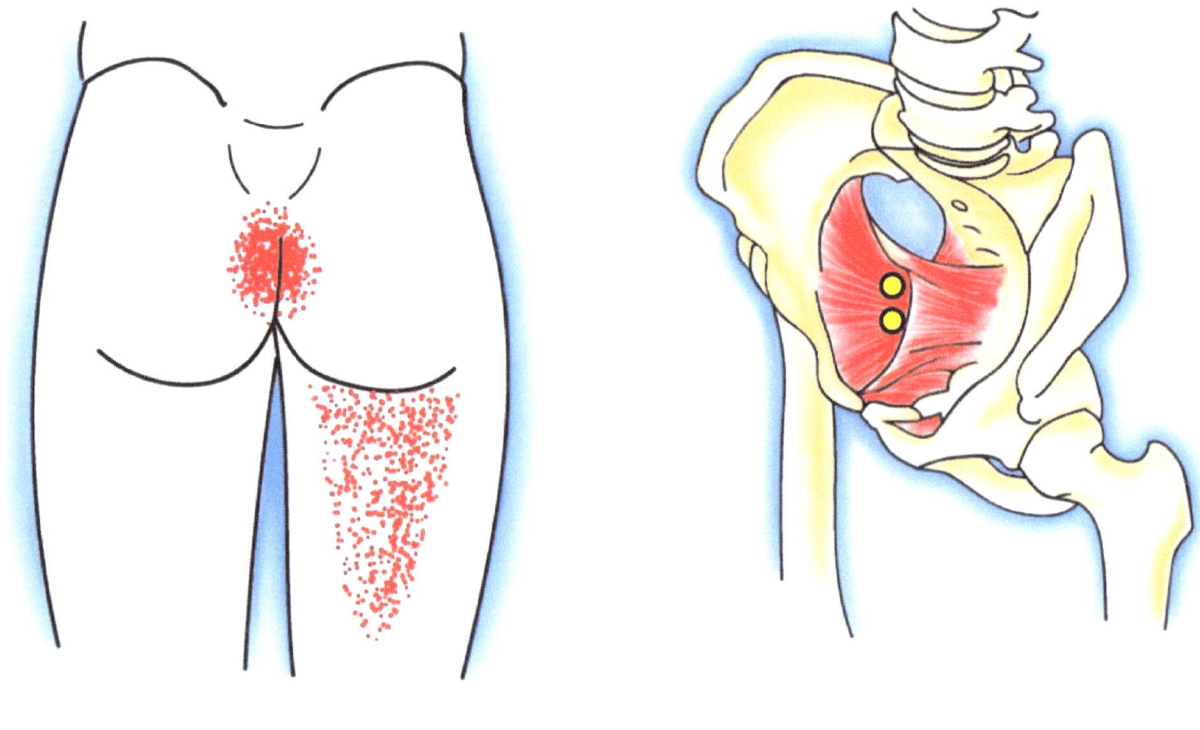

Figure 7.11A   Figure 7.11B

Obturator Internus muscle (Figure 7.11B) trigger points can cause pain in the anal region and down the back of the leg (Figure 7.11A). Symptoms can include painful bowel movements, and painful sex (notably during entry), and a feeling of fullness in the rectum.[23]

---

[23] (Travell, MD & Simons MD, Myofascial Pain and Dysfunction. The Trigger Point Manual. The Lower Extremities., 1992)

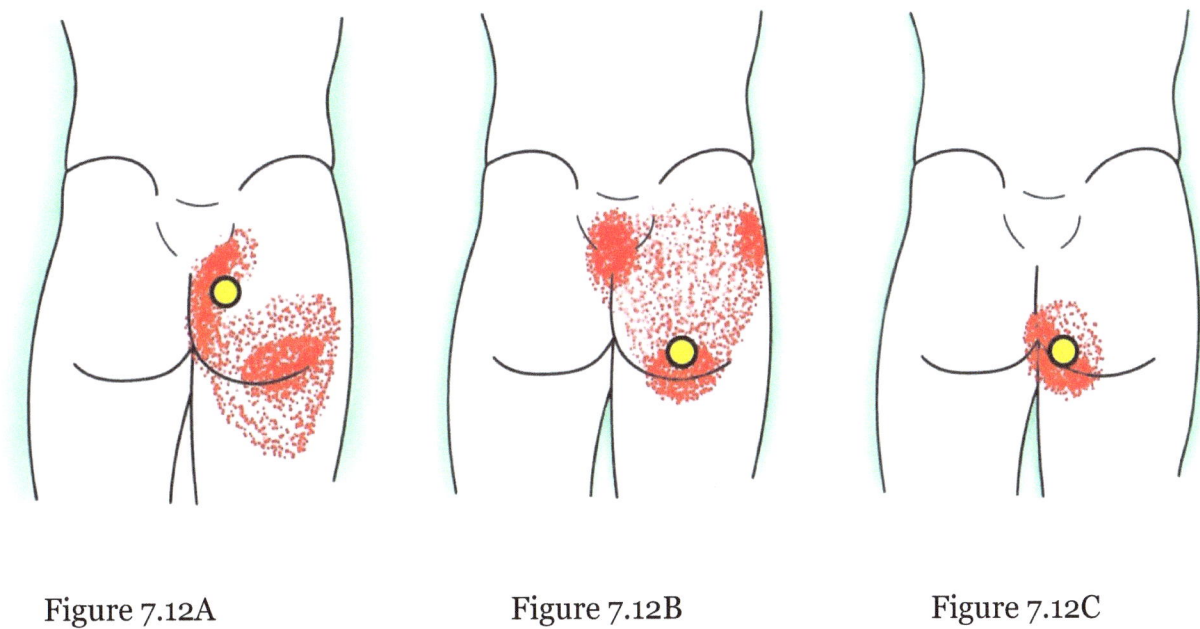

Figure 7.12A   Figure 7.12B   Figure 7.12C

Gluteus Maximus trigger points (Figure 7.12A, Figure 7.12B, and Figure 7.12C) refer pain and tenderness to the sacrum region, down to the gluteal fold and behind the thigh, along the ilium and into the coccyx.[24]

---

[24] (Travell, MD & Simons MD, Myofascial Pain and Dysfunction. The Trigger Point Manual. The Lower Extremities., 1992)

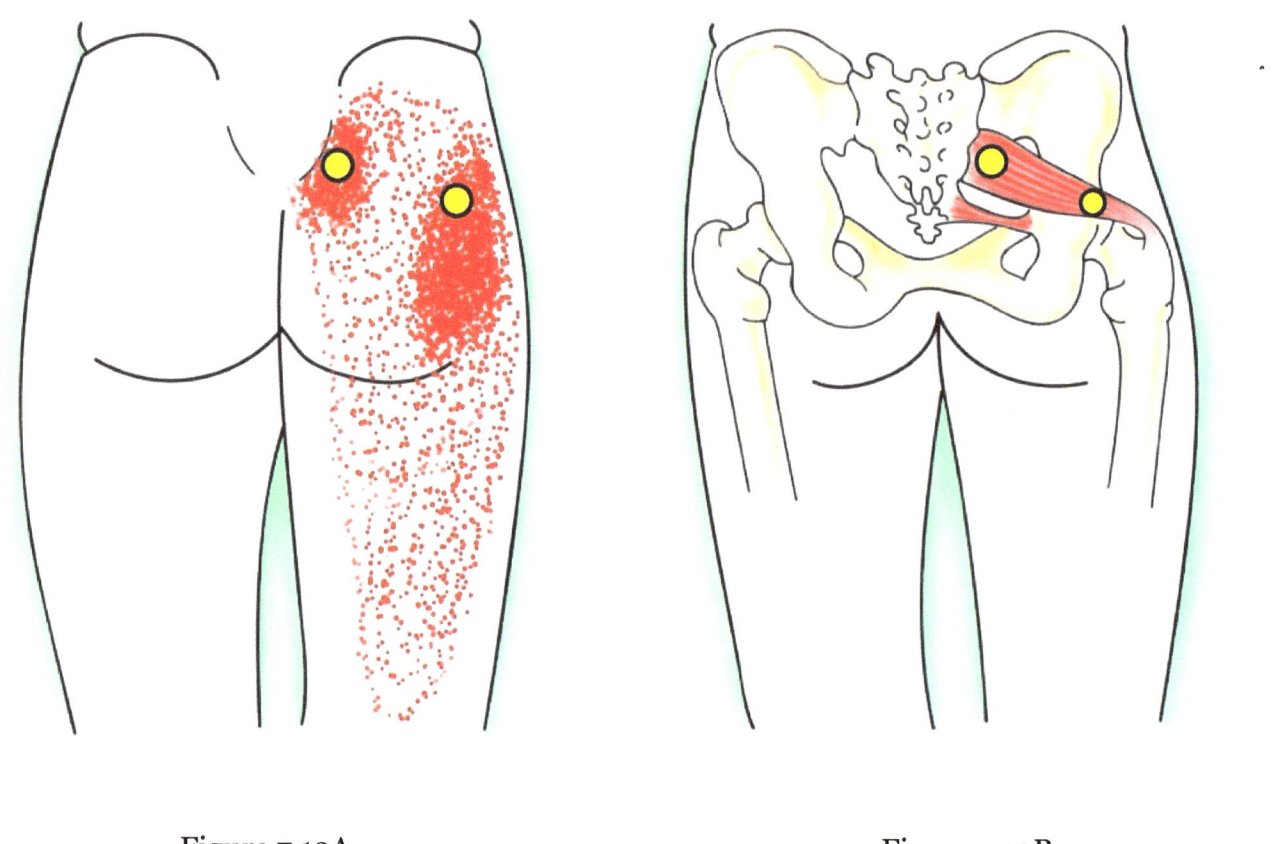

Figure 7.13A Figure 7.13B

Piriformis muscle trigger points (Figure 7.13B) refer pain primarily into the sacroiliac region, to the glute and down the back of the thigh (Figure 7.13A).[25]

---

[25] (Travell, MD & Simons MD, Myofascial Pain and Dysfunction. The Trigger Point Manual. The Lower Extremities., 1992)

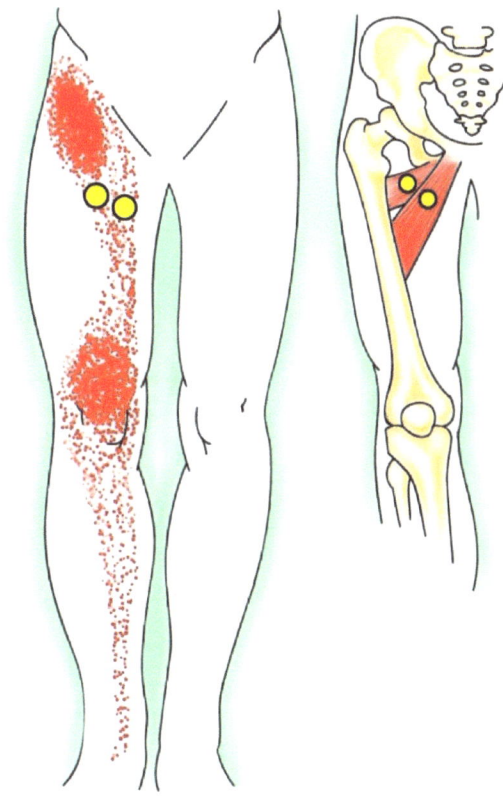

Figure 7.14A   Figure 7.14B

Abductor Brevis trigger points (Figure 7.14B) refer pain into the groin, and down to the knee and medial region of lower leg (Figure 7.14A). This pain is described as a deep groin pain, often felt like a pelvic pain, however the patient cannot pinpoint an exact spot where the pain is in the pelvis.[26]

---

[26] (Travell, MD & Simons MD, Myofascial Pain and Dysfunction. The Trigger Point Manual. The Lower Extremities., 1992)

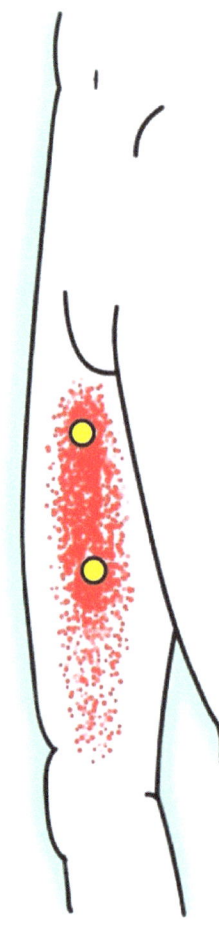

Figure 7.15

Gracilis muscle trigger points (Figure 7.15) can cause a constant burning pain down the inside of the leg.[27]

---

[27] (Travell, MD & Simons MD, Myofascial Pain and Dysfunction. The Trigger Point Manual. The Lower Extremities., 1992)

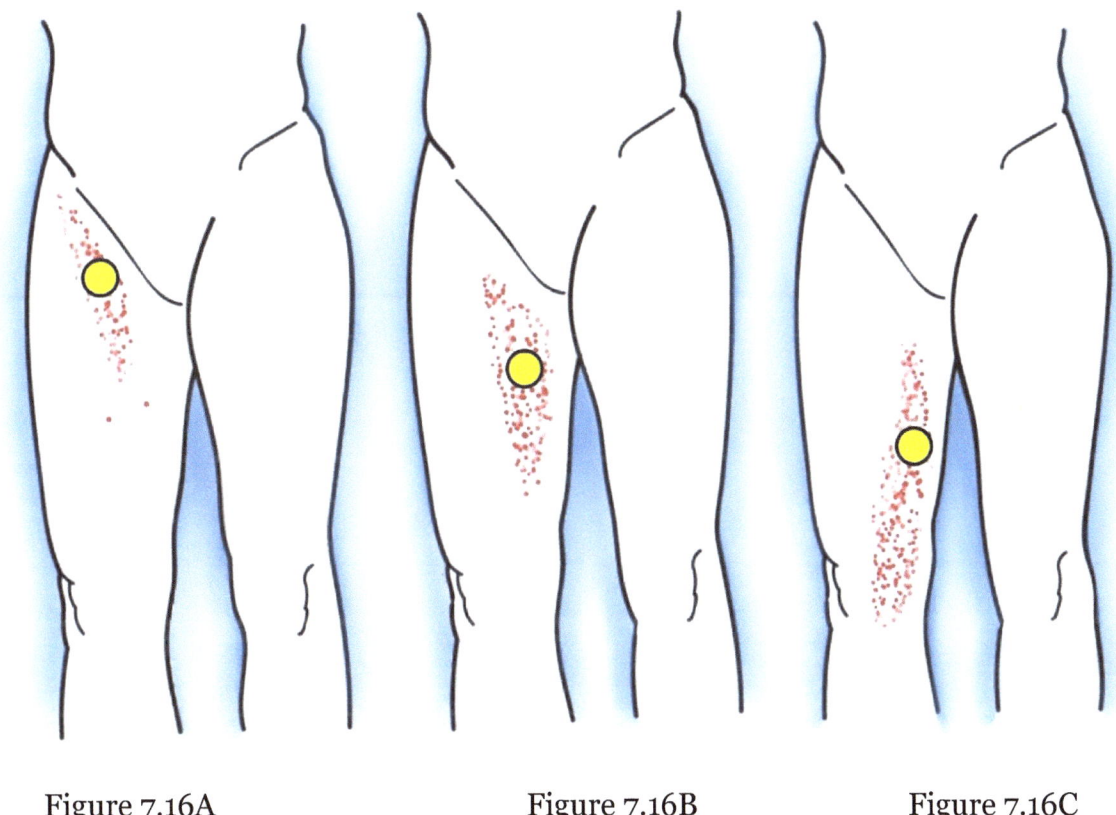

Figure 7.16A Figure 7.16B Figure 7.16C

Sartorius muscle trigger points can be found from the front of the pelvis down the inside of the leg (Figure 7.16A, Figure 7.16B, and Figure 7.16C). The pain can radiate along the muscle and into the inner knee. [28]

---

[28] (Travell, MD & Simons MD, Myofascial Pain and Dysfunction. The Trigger Point Manual. The Lower Extremities., 1992)

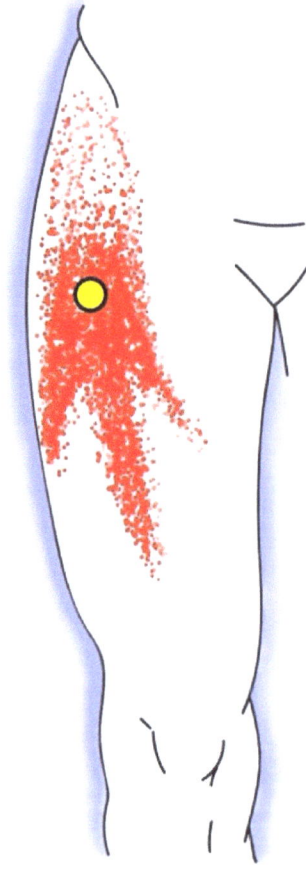

Figure 7.17

Vastus Intermedius muscle trigger points (Figure 7.17) refer pain from down the center of the thigh to mid-thigh.[29]

---

[29] (Travell, MD & Simons MD, Myofascial Pain and Dysfunction. The Trigger Point Manual. The Lower Extremities., 1992)

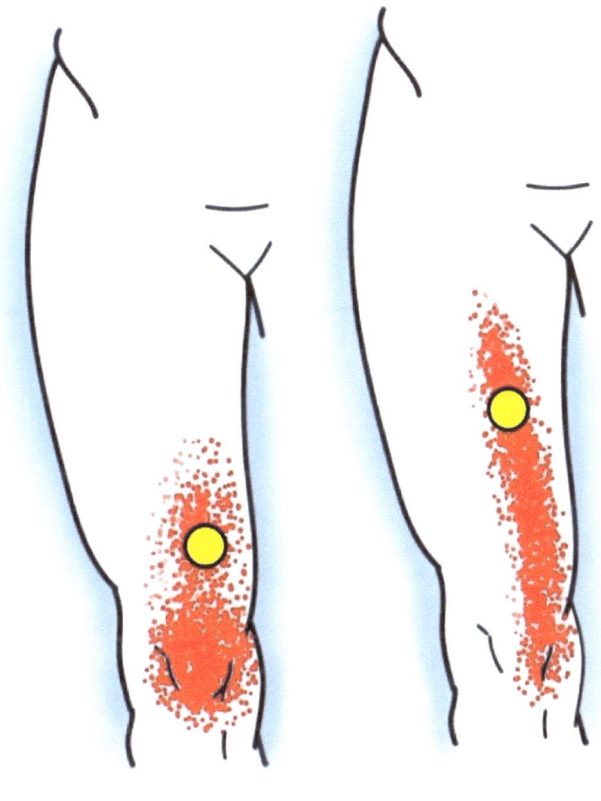

Figure 7.18A   Figure 7.18B

Vastus Medialis muscle trigger points (Figure 7.18A, and Figure 7.18B) can cause pain down the front of the thigh (Figure 7.18B) and into the knee (Figure 7.18A). These trigger points can refer an aching pain into the front of the knee and thigh.[30]

---

[30] (Travell, MD & Simons MD, Myofascial Pain and Dysfunction. The Trigger Point Manual. The Lower Extremities., 1992)

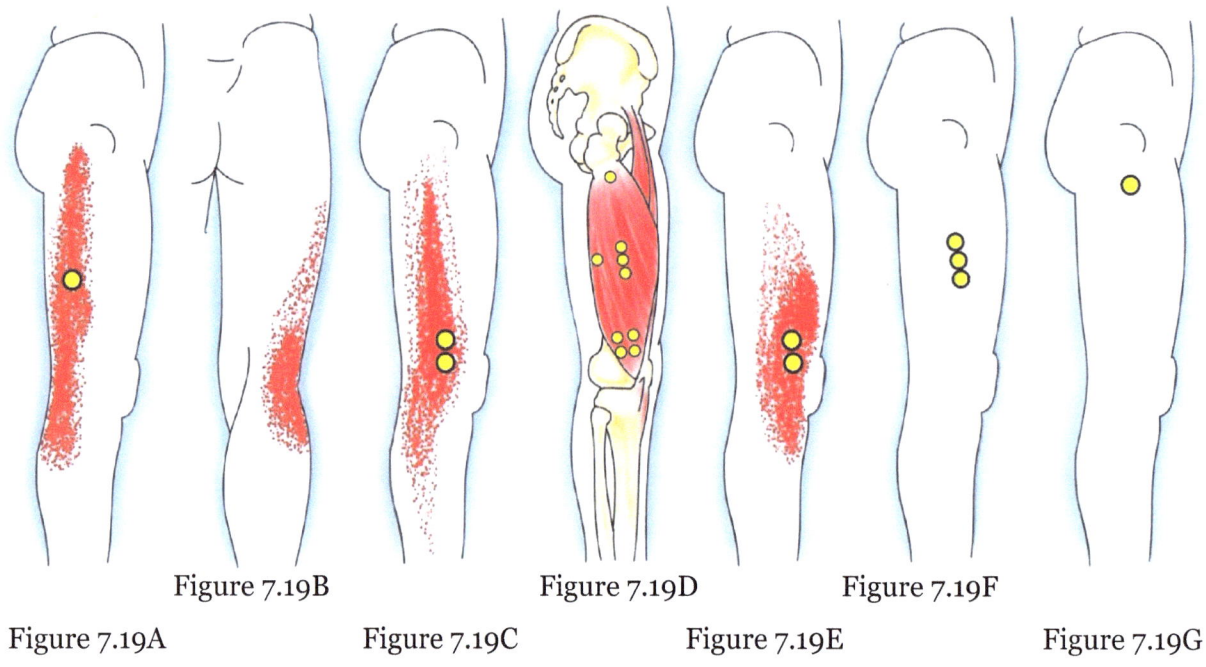

Figure 7.19A
Figure 7.19B
Figure 7.19C
Figure 7.19D
Figure 7.19E
Figure 7.19F
Figure 7.19G

Vastus Lateralis muscles has various sites of trigger points (Figure 7.19D). This pain can be felt along the side of the leg (Figure 7.19A, Figure 7.19B, and Figure 7.19C) and into the outer knee (Figure 7.19E).[31]

---

[31] (Travell, MD & Simons MD, Myofascial Pain and Dysfunction. The Trigger Point Manual. The Lower Extremities., 1992)

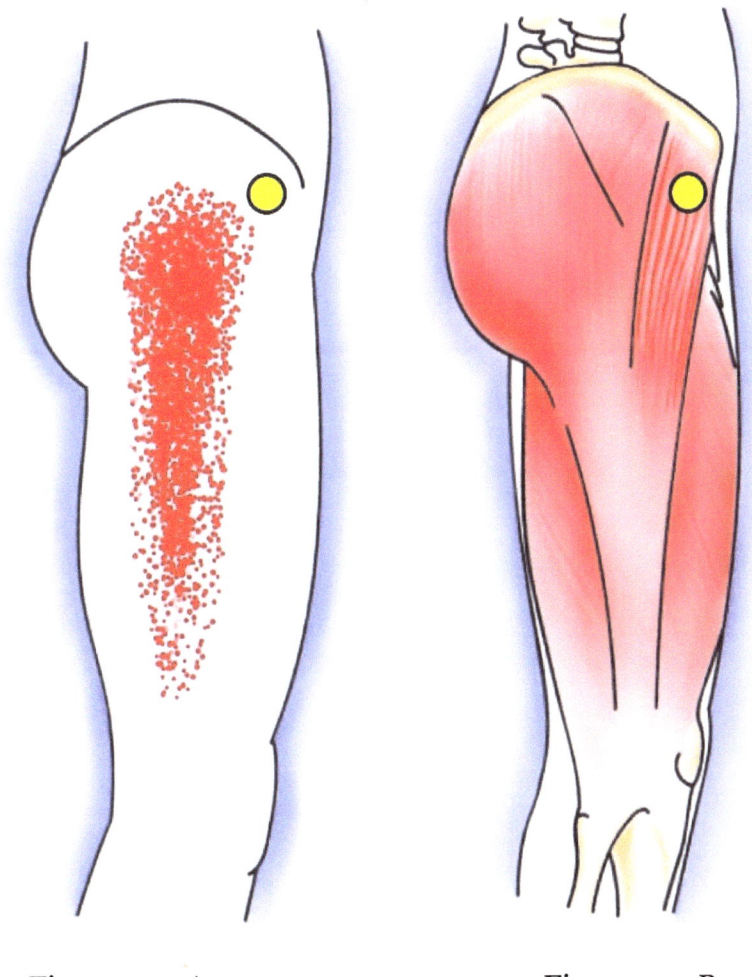

Figure 7.20A   Figure 7.20B

Tensor Fasciae Latae (TFL) muscle trigger points (Figure 7.20B) refer pain into the hip and down the side thigh (Figure 7.20A).[32]

---

[32] (Travell, MD & Simons MD, Myofascial Pain and Dysfunction. The Trigger Point Manual. The Lower Extremities., 1992)

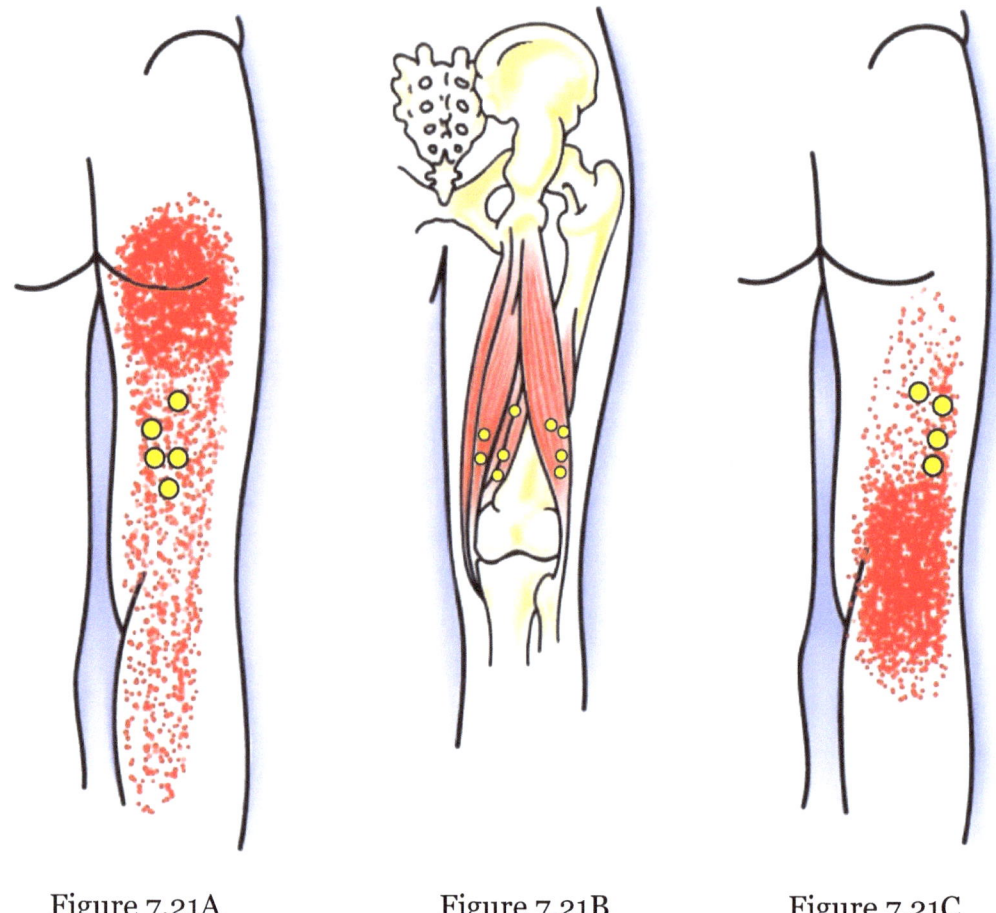

Figure 7.21A   Figure 7.21B   Figure 7.21C

Hamstring muscles have various sites trigger points that can develop (Figure 7.21B). Referred pain can be felt from the lower buttocks and back of the thigh all the way down to the back of the calf muscle (Figure 7.21A). Referred pain can also be felt in the back of the knee (Figure 7.21C). This pain gets worse when walking.[33]

---

[33] (Travell, MD & Simons MD, Myofascial Pain and Dysfunction. The Trigger Point Manual. The Lower Extremities., 1992)

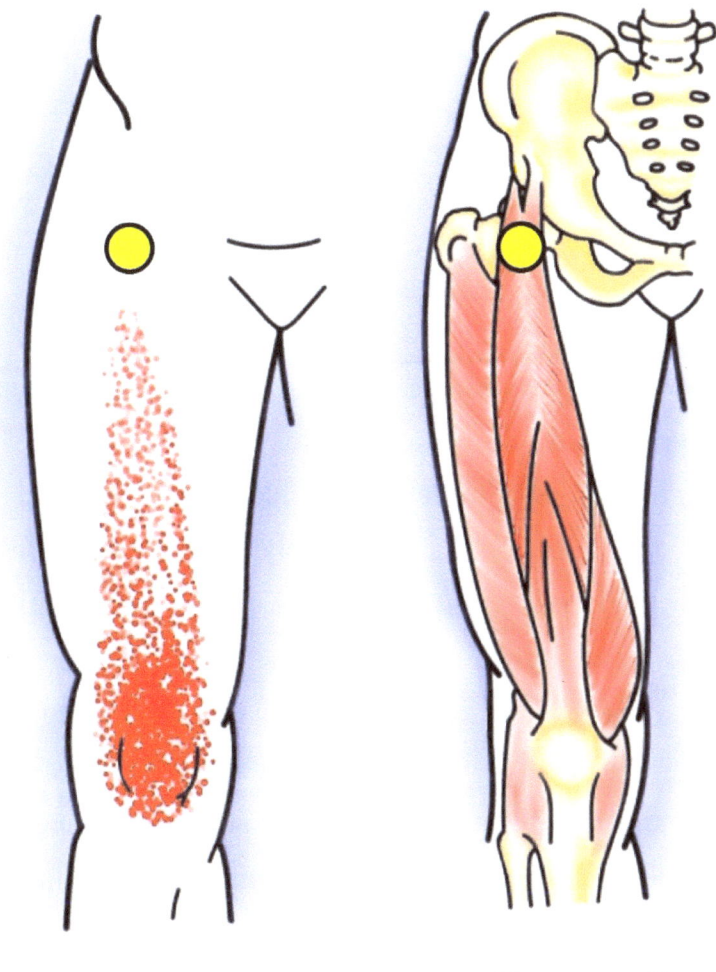

Figure 7.22A Figure 7.22B

Rectus Femoris muscle trigger point (Figure 7.22B) refers pain down the front of thigh into the knee (Figure 7.22A).[34]

---

[34] (Travell, MD & Simons MD, Myofascial Pain and Dysfunction. The Trigger Point Manual. The Lower Extremities., 1992)

How Trigger Point Therapy Works:

To release a trigger point, you need to compress and hold the point. This temporarily blocks the blood flow to the trigger point. This technique forces the blood and lymph out of the area and signals the trigger point to release. This is called applying ischemic compression, and it can be done using a few different techniques. I describe some helpful ones here.

Trigger point balls

There are several different balls you can use, each a different density (firmness). Start with a massage ball until the trigger point releases a little and the pain lessens. Then try a tennis ball, and lastly a lacrosse ball if the trigger point remains. I like to start out with a massage ball which has more give, because your trigger points are probably very sensitive. Begin by looking at the map of different bodies with trigger points and figure out where your trigger points are. For example, the one on the front of your thigh. Look at the picture of the muscles, the yellow O's mark the trigger points and the different red colors show where you would be feeling pain. Find one that matches where you're feeling pain, then feel with your hand over the area to try to feel where that little nodule is. In the beginning, when you first start trigger point therapy, you may not be able to feel the nodule, because your whole leg is going to be painful. If that's the case, and you can't feel it, it's okay. Put the ball right where you *think* the trigger point would be, and then lie on the ball. While you are laying on the ball compressing your trigger point, do the diaphragmatic breathing. This will help keep your pelvic floor relaxed during the trigger point therapy. You do not want the pelvic floor to go into a clenching mode. Roll around, back and forth, on the trigger point, massaging with the ball. You need to be able to breathe through this. If it is too intense (painful), don't start directly on the trigger point. Start to the side of it, and gently roll onto the trigger point until you can stand the direct pressure. If you go too hard you won't be able to breathe, and that will put you into a clenching (or guarding) state. It is very important that you avoid clenching, so roll around and breathe. Do this for a full minute and move on to the next trigger point. If you do this every day, you'll notice that your pain levels in those areas start to lessen. The pain area will start to shrink. When that trigger point isn't so sensitive, then move to a ball that's a little harder, like a tennis ball, and repeat the exercise. After the tennis ball, you can move to a lacrosse ball to release the last of the trigger point and receive complete relief.

Massage Therapy

Massage therapy is very effective for relieving trigger points. It's important that you go to somebody who knows how to work with trigger points. Someone who uses slow, consistent pressure on the trigger points. There are different massage techniques that are not as painful as others. For example, rocking and shaking, trigger point work with breath, and so on. A deep tissue massage may not be the best technique, as it can go too deep, causing you to clench. It is very important the massage therapist does not go past your comfortable pain threshold levels, as this will do more harm than good. The process will be slow, but more effective in the long run, if you can avoid flare-ups with therapy. Always speak up if the pressure level is making it difficult to remain relaxed, especially in your pelvic floor. If you cannot take comfortable breaths, it is too deep. The process will be slow, but more effective in the long run, if you can avoid flare-ups with therapy. Doing your diaphragmatic breathing during your massage can help keep your pelvic floor relaxed, thereby encouraging new postural patterns.

Finding a good, qualified, massage therapist becomes essential. I found it helpful to ask around and get a referral from a friend. You want somebody who knows how work with trigger points and can put you on some type of plan. You're going to need more than one massage. Once a week would be great, twice a week is okay too, with enough rest and healing days between sessions. You just don't want to go so often that you're sore from the previous massage.

Cupping

This is an effective way to work on trigger points, and I've used it with success. Cupping draws blood and lymph from a trigger point through the application of negative pressure. It is like getting massage from the inside out. Note! There will be bruising on your skin after.

If you watched the 2016 Summer Olympics with swimmer Michael Phelps, you may have noticed purple circles around his shoulders and back. With each event, he had more purple circles on him. He was getting cupped as part of his recovery routine, to help to relieve the muscles he strained during a race, and quickly prepare for the next race. You can either get cupping done from an acupuncturist, or you can do it at home. You can buy a cupping kit from various websites that sell products online. The one that I've used has a handle, you put the cup on the trigger point, and engage the hand pump on the cup to suck the air out. Again, you will get red marks on your skin. This is not permanent, and the marks will disappear within a week. I found it best to apply a thin layer of oil or cream to the skin first, this makes for a good seal when the cups are applied. You can slightly pump it once the cup is in place to gently move the fluids around more. Put one cup over a trigger point, and more cups on the sore muscles the trigger point radiates to. This will help relieve the symptomatic tight muscles as well as the trigger point.

Dry Needling

According to the Journal of Manual & Manipulative Therapy, dry needling reverses some aspects of central sensitization. Central sensitization is a state of the nervous system associated with chronic pain, where the nervous system has constant elevated sensitiveness. Dry needling reduces local and referred pain, improves range of motion and muscle activation pattern, and alters the chemical environment of trigger points[35].

I have found dry needling to be the most effective technique for addressing trigger points. Note that this is not acupuncture. Dry needling is performed by a Chiropractor, Physical Therapist, Nurse, MD or Acupuncturist, who has had training in the technique of dry needling.

Through my research, I had the honor of interviewing Dr. Edward Cremata. He has a vast knowledge of trigger point therapy and dry needling. Dr. Cremata has practiced chiropractic for 36 years and has spent 25 years teaching in the field. He has a bachelor's degree in nursing and is a licensed Registered Nurse (RN).

Dr. Cremata is an expert in the field of trigger point therapy, and personally helped me to reduce and eliminate the trigger points I had that were contributing to my own CPP. I asked him to share with me what he knows of trigger points and how the therapy works.

He typically sees patients with CPP who have trigger points in the low back, glutes, internal pelvic, coccygeal, and lower extremities. They either have latent trigger points where the pain is locally restricted, or active ones that are hot, painful and refer pain to other regions. The trigger point is a knotty region where the muscle is constricted perpetually, stopping the muscle from functioning correctly. The trigger point keeps constant, abnormal stress on the muscle. Dr. Cremata uses a therapy known as 'dry needling' to reduce and eliminate these trigger points. This is the process by which a thin needle (like an acupuncture needle) is inserted directly into

---

[35] (Dommerholt, 2011)

the heart of the trigger point, then rotated. This breaks up the knot, releasing the muscle. Typically, people need 5 – 7 sessions for noticeable results[36].

It's important to identify the exact trigger point so you can be precise. Putting a bunch of needles in a painful region, hoping to find a trigger point is not going to work. Dr. Cremata warns against having this procedure done by someone other than a trained professional, if the needle is too long, it might puncture a vital organ (like a lung when working on trigger points in the back) or a tendon (when working on trigger points around an ankle). This can have a devastating impact. The needle must be inserted directly into the trigger point in a muscle, using alcohol for sterilization, and the right protocol for the area and type of trigger point.

Dry needling is a safe and effective process when done by a competent practitioner. Dr. Cremata says it's imperative you find a trained professional licensed to do a medical procedure that penetrates the skin and who knows the correct protocol. You can find someone in your area by reaching out to educational institutes who teach it.

Dry needling is a useful technique for everyone who has trigger points. Stretching alone will not release a tight muscle if trigger points are present. If done correctly, dry needling incorporated into my Pelvic Pain Program can be an important part of the healing solution. It was for me.

Magnesium Supplementation

According to The National Academy of Science, a majority of Americans are magnesium deficient and this can lead to many health problems[37]. Magnesium regulates 325 enzymes to enable your

---

[36] (Cremata DC RN, 2018)
[37] (Universal Health Institute)

body to function optimally. Magnesium helps improve nerve and muscle function, reduces inflammation, increases oxygenation, and improves blood flow. Magnesium deficiency may be a contributor to many common women's health conditions, including PMS, hormonal migraines, endometriosis, and polycystic ovarian syndrome. You can see why getting adequate magnesium is important if you have chronic pelvic pain! Get your blood work done by your primary physician to see if you are low in magnesium.

Some suggestions from doctors to boost your body's magnesium levels include, eating foods high in magnesium, such as avocados, seeds and leafy greens, supplementation (ask your chiropractor or physician which ones), and soaking in Epsom salt[38].

Taking a warm Epsom salt bath can help your pelvic floor relax during your soak. This is perfect to do before bedtime to help you sleep. Our bodies heal when we sleep, so the better you sleep, the better your body can heal. Performing slow diaphragmatic breathing during your soak can also help de-stress your body and mind. I understand the frustration, anger, and sadness that accompanies chronic pelvic pain. Sometimes, just taking a moment for you is necessary to change your perspective and improve your mood. To adjust your thinking from just surviving to thriving.

The Endocannabinoid System

We have different systems in our body. The Circulatory System, Digestive System, Endocrine System, Lymphatic System (Immune System), Muscular System, Nervous System, and Renal System (Urinary, Excretory System), Reproductive System, Respiratory System, Skeletal System

---

[38] (Waring, Dr R H, 2015)

and the Endocannabinoid System (ECS). As a chiropractor I am primarily focused on the Nervous System, but I knew my CPP involved more that this system alone. I began to research other systems which may be involved with my pain. This led me to learn about the Endocannabinoid System (ECS). This major system was discovered in 1992 by Dr. Mechoulam, of Hebrew University in Jerusalem, Israel. I was surprised to learn of this system, it was new information to me! Here is just a little information about this system and what does and why it matters for healing.

The purpose of the ECS is to maintain the delicate balance that naturally occurs in our body. The ECS is composed of receptor sites and endogenous (made in our body) endocannabinoids. These receptors are found throughout our body, in the brain, organs, glands, connective tissue, and immune cells. The ECS helps to regulate the physiological systems within our body responsible for pain-sensation, mood, memory, appetite, and more. I was curious to see if boosting this system would help me. Our bodies naturally make our own endocannabinoids which support the ECS, but I discovered we can also take supplementation to boost it.

Cannabinoids

There are three distinct cannabinoids that stimulate these receptors in our body. The one discussed above is found naturally occurring in our own body, this is the endogenous cannabinoids. The next one is engineered in a lab and is known as synthetic cannabinoids. The last one is naturally produced by plants, known as phytocannabinoids.

Plants with naturally occurring phytocannabinoids, or those that have properties similar to the effect of phytocannabinoids (with varying degrees of efficacy), are the following:

- Coneflower (Echinacea)
- Electric Daisy (Acmella Oleracea)
- Helichrysum Umbraculigerum
- Liverwort (Radula Marginata)
- Black Pepper (Piper Nigrum)
- Chocolate (Theobroma Cacao)
- Chinese Rhododendron
- Kava (Piper Methysticum)
- Cannabis (Hemp and Marijuana)

Cannabis has two families, think of them as cousins. The first is the Hemp family of plants containing approximately 500 compounds. Of these, approximately 100 are phytocannabinoids (THC and CBD included), 100 are terpenoids and the remainder are flavonoids, fatty acids, and enzymes. These all work together in a complementary way, and they play an important role. The other family is Marijuana. There are a couple of substantial differences in these two subspecies. Most notably, the appearance, and the amount of THC secreted. Hemp produces only trace amounts (0.3%) THC (this is non-psychoactive) and Marijuana contains anywhere from 6 – 20% of THC (this is extremely psychoactive).

Hemp is legal in all states, however, at the time of this book, some states are still trying to work out the legal differences between hemp and marijuana. By definition, hemp is legal as long as it stays true to the definition, which is non-psychoactive, or less than or equal to 0.3% of THC.

I encourage you do your own research on the ECS and cannabinoids to make an educated decision if this is something right for you. Here are some useful articles to get you started.

Linking the Endocannabinoid System with modulation of pain and inflammation
www.ncbi.nlm.nih.gov/pmc/articles/PMC3820295/

Topically applied cannabidiol gel eased osteoarthritis pain

https://www.ncbi.nlm.nih.gov/pmc/articles/PMC4851925/

Early Phase inflammation by cannabidiol prevents pain and nerve damage

https://www.ncbi.nlm.nih.gov/pmc/articles/PMC5690292/

Chapter 8

Taking Back Your Power

PHASE 4: Re-Balancing Your Core Unit

The Core Unit muscles are unique in that they anticipate motion (sensorimotor), and when working correctly, they fire before the start of movement, and maintain a low-grade contraction throughout all motion activities. They form a stable inner mechanism for the spine and allow the outer unit to move the body around this stable structure. When there is dysfunction in the unit, you experience muscle chaos. The core unit is the foundation of stability for the rest of the body. Each muscle is linked intimately through this sensorimotor system. When you have pelvic dysfunction, there will be other issues that follow, groin strains, low back pain, anterior knee pain, and so on.

The Core Unit consists of four muscles Figure 8.1

- Diaphragm
- Multifidus
- Transversus Abdominal (TrA)
- Pelvic Floor

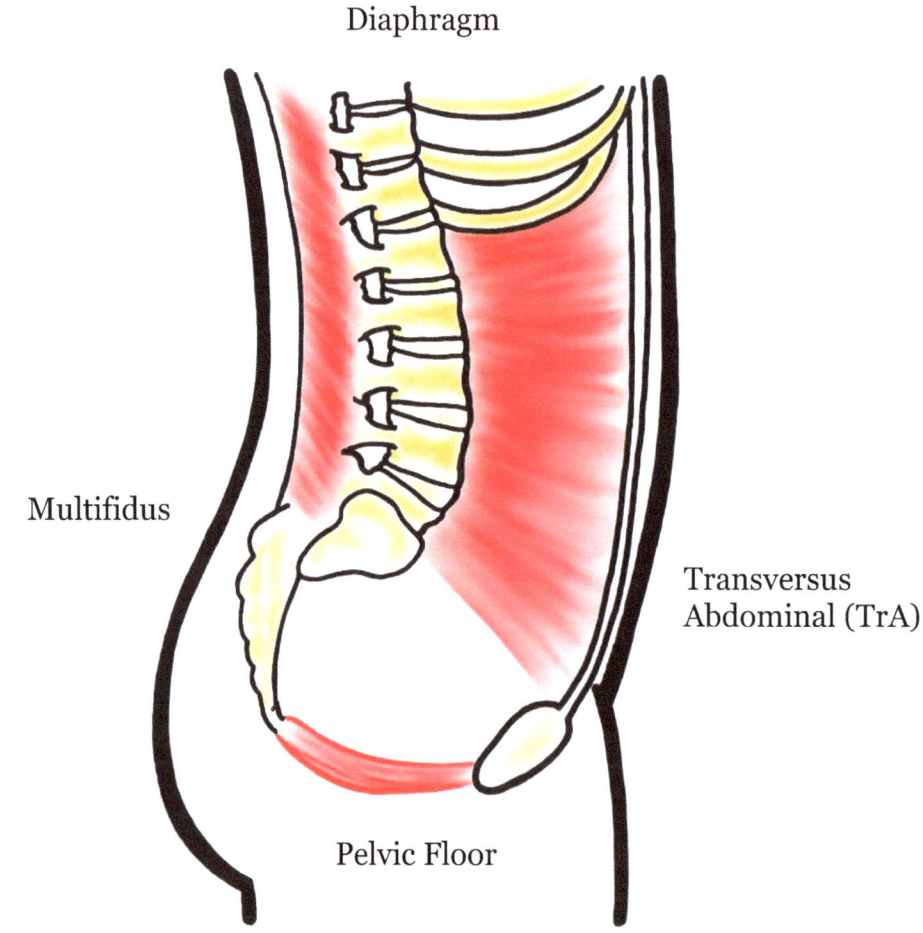

Figure 8.1

BALANCED CORE Muscles   IMBALANCED CORE Muscles

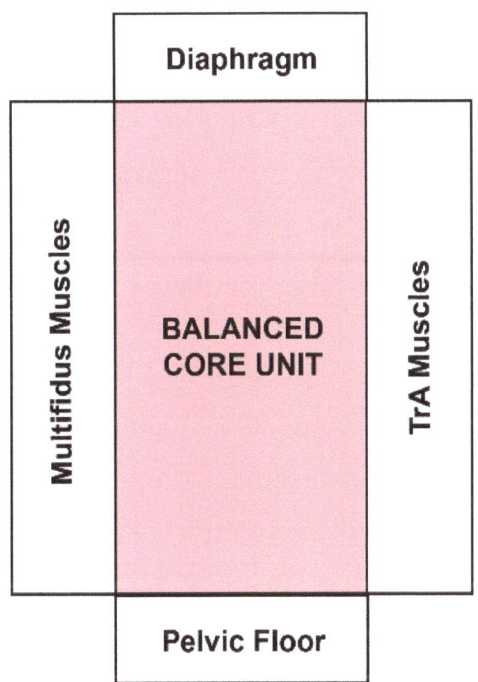 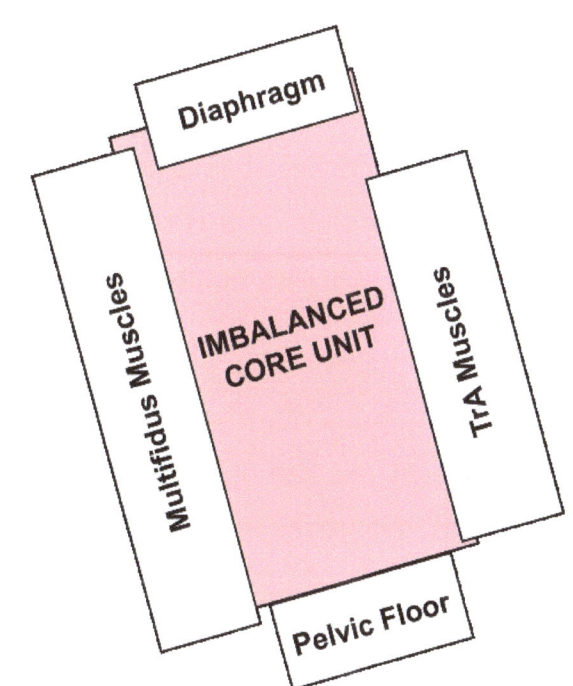

Side Effects of Imbalanced Core Unit

- Shallow Breathing
- TrA shut down or increased tone
- Shortened Pelvic Floor, increased tone
- Some Multifidi not firing

Re-balancing your Core Unit

Now that you know how to relax your pelvic floor, and can identify clenching through the breathing exercises, you are ready for the next phase.

When people think of working out their core, the 'go-to' exercises are planks or crunches. However, planks and crunches should be avoided when you have pelvic floor weakness. The pelvic floor is the weakest link in the core unit and these types of exercises can easily overload a weakened pelvic floor and drive you into another flare-up.

This is a key point to understand in order to avoid flare-ups from working out when your inner unit is not functioning properly. If you are like me, I was tired of not being able to do physical activities, so I worked out through the pain, creating many more muscular compensatory patterns, which lead to more trigger points, and just increased my pain.

These first exercises are designed to identify, and correct, this imbalance and to start your core unit functioning properly. DO NOT move on to the next phase of exercises until you have these muscles working together. That is, move on when you can do the exercises easily, and with little thought.

Diaphragm Breathing - Warm Up

Reps: 5

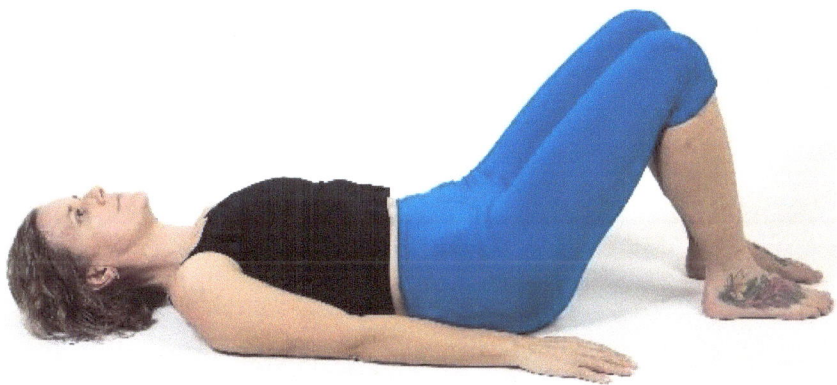

Position: Lay on your back, with both legs bent, and your feet on the ground.

Movement: Breathe deeply into your belly, without breathing into your chest.

** This is to ensure you are not clenching whilst doing these strengthening exercises.

(Pelvic Floor Activation is necessary to strengthen these other muscles.)

Transversus Abdominal Muscles (TrA) – Turning Them On

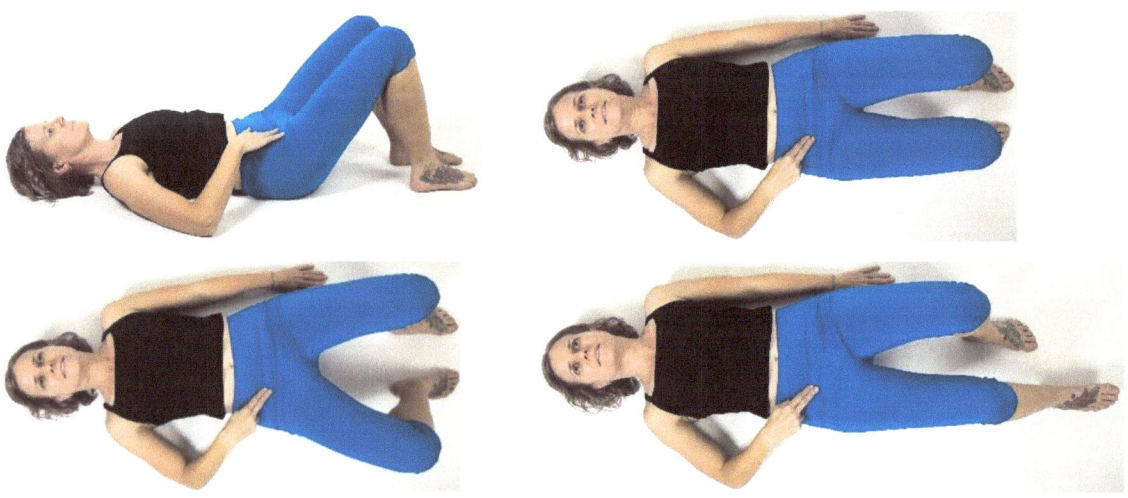

Position: Lay on your back, with both legs bent, and your feet on the ground. Using your fingertips, locate the inside front corners of your pelvis, 1" towards midline (belly button) and 1" down. Do one side at a time.

Movement: Contract your pelvic floor (tighten your lower abs, just below your finger). You should feel that muscle underneath your fingertips pop up. If you do not feel the muscle under your finger, allow the leg on the same side to open slightly towards the floor. This is similar to the adductor stretch, while also contracting your pelvic floor. That muscle should pop up with the increased stress. Eventually you will get to the place where you can contract the TrA without having to move the leg. Repeat on the other side.

**Goal: Ability to activate the TrA in isolation (without pelvic floor contraction).
*** Advanced: While contracting TrA, slightly let the heel of your foot on the same side drag on the floor, away from your pelvis. This will gently challenge your TrA, to help strengthen it.

Multifidus Muscles

The Multifidus muscles can shut down from just one minor impact to the low back. You may have had an issue in this area long before you experienced pelvic pain. The Multifidus are small muscles that stabilize the spine. It is common for people with pelvic floor dysfunction to eventually get low back pain. These muscles are in the deepest layer of your back. You cannot strengthen these muscles by working out in the gym. Turning them on is quite easy, and yet at the same time, challenging.

You will need someone to help you identify which ones are shut down, so you can consciously turn them back on.

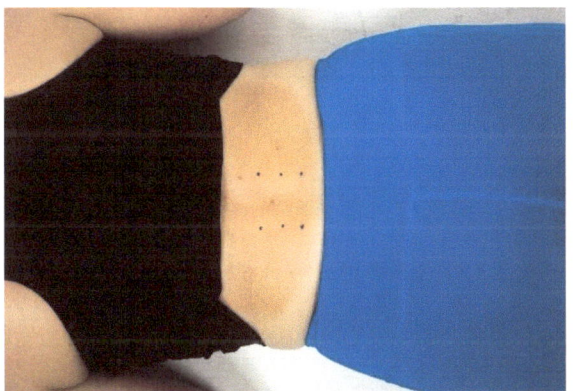 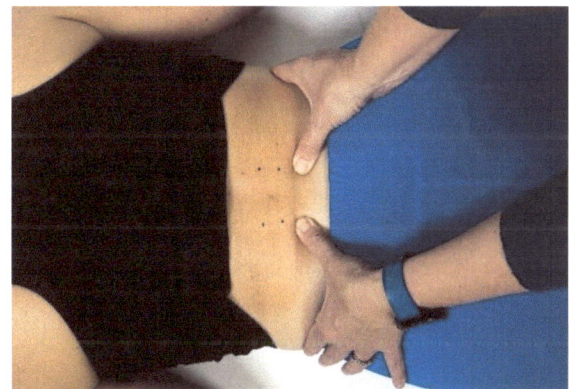

Instruction for contracting muscles: Under your partner's thumb, try to push their thumb up or off your back. This will help you isolate the weak Multifidus muscle to turn it on.

Tra and Multifidus Together

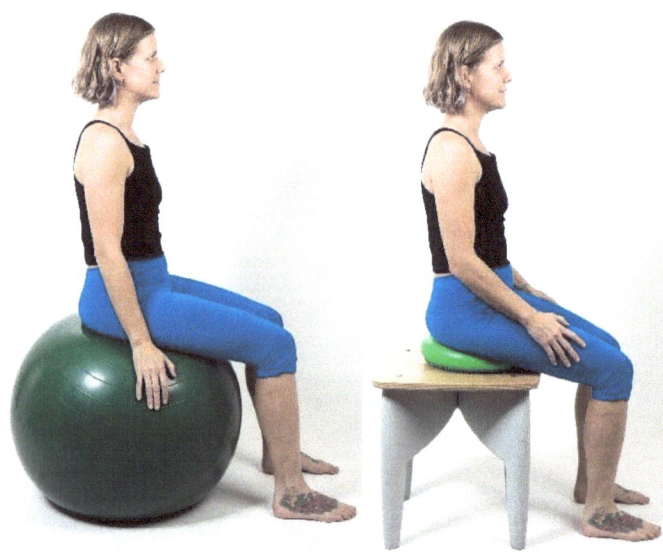

Position: Sit on a ball, or chair if you do not have a stability ball

Movement: Slowly tighten your TrA and Multifidus together. Try to breathe while holding them both tight. When you can breathe comfortably, lift one foot (as though kicking a ball, this is to put a stress on the core unit, but not to fire your hip flexors). This will begin to re-educate your TrA and Multifidus to contract with motion.

Once you have reactivated all core muscles, you can begin to re-educate them to function together, as they were meant to do. This exercise works with your neurology feedback loop. This is nerve feedback from your feet, up to your brain, and back to your feet; a communication loop.

Balance Stand and Re-educate the Core

Position: Use a stool or wall initially to help with balance, but quickly learn to balance without it.
Stand on the disc, feet hip-width apart.

Movement: Initially: Maintain your balance for one minute. Once your balance improves: Rock onto the balls of your feet and back to the heels of your feet. Continue the motion for 30 seconds – to one minute. You will be working your hips and thighs, while re-educating your core to automatically engage.

Note - do not clench. Your core should engage automatically, without you physically tightening it. You should not be keeping yourself rigid when balancing. Allow your body to sway naturally as you try to stand on the disc.

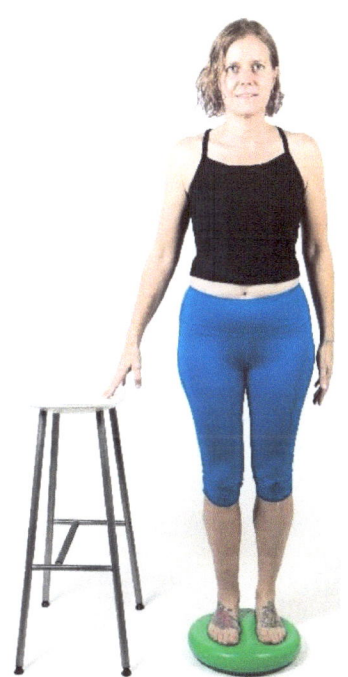

Chapter 9

Strengthening and Stretching

Phase V: Let's Get Moving!

This is the most important phase. Now that you are feeling better, and have less pain with movement, it is time to strengthen the muscles that have become weakened from CPP. When you have an imbalance in the pelvic stabilizers, you will continue to have flare-ups and irritate your trigger points. With balanced pelvic stabilizers, there will be fewer flare-ups and irritated trigger points.

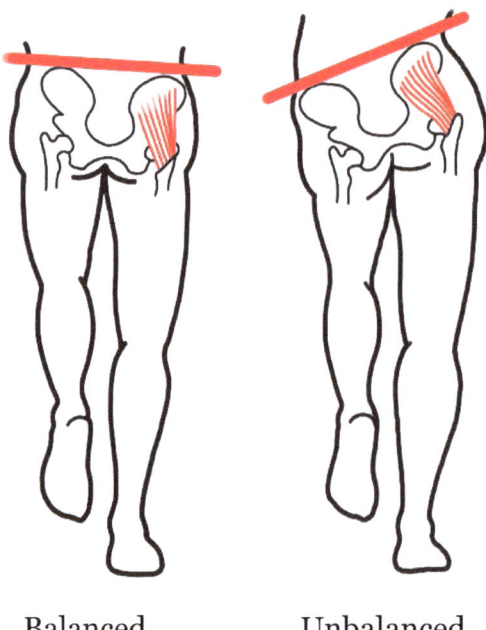

Balanced   Unbalanced

Strengthening

Bridges

Reps: Start with slow repetitions, and progress to holds from 2-10 seconds

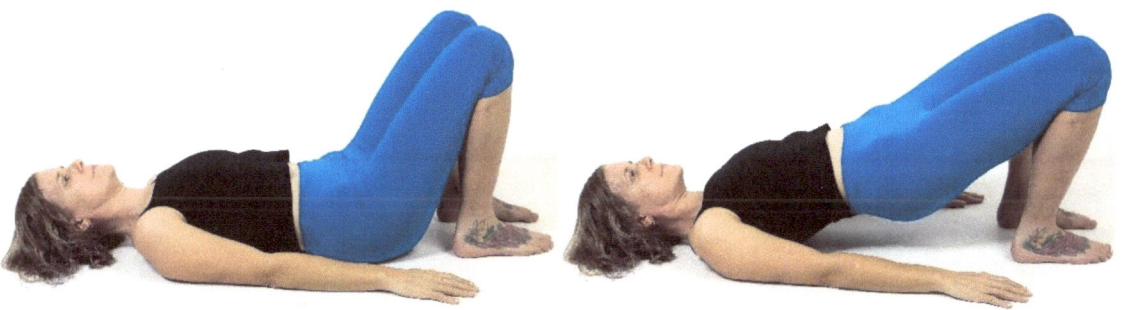

Position: Lie on back, with knees bent, feet planted on the floor.

Movement: Maintain core stability and keep your spine straight, while contracting the glute muscles. Raise your buttocks from the floor, until your hips are in line with your shoulders and knees.

**Key points: Take deep diaphragmatic breaths throughout. Make sure when you rest between reps, you are not clenching.

Clams

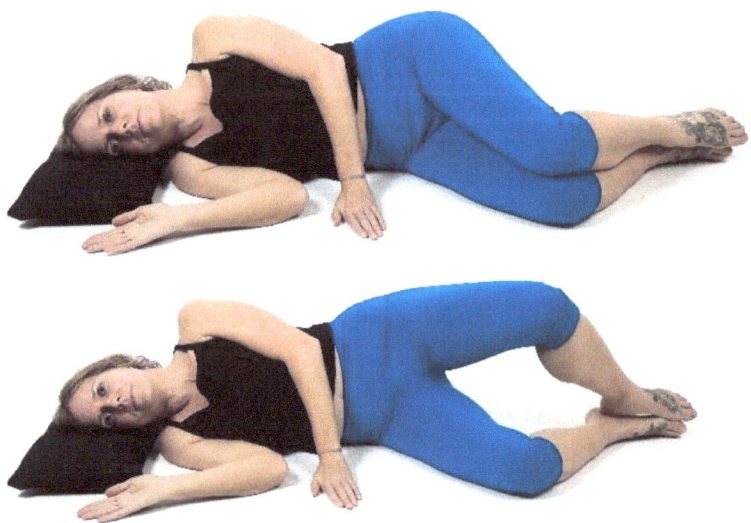

Position: Lie on your side (put a pillow your under head for comfort) with your knees bent.

Movement: Contract the core muscles and pull your belly button towards your spine. Then, keeping your ankles together, and your spine still, raise the top of one knee.

Key Point: Do not allow your body to lean.

Hip Internal Rotators

Reps: Start out slowly, and progress to holds from 2-10 seconds

Position: Sit on the edge of a chair, with your legs over the edge. Loop a stretching strap or belt around your ankles, keep your knees bent at a right angle. Put a ball or pillow between your knees.

Movement: Pull your ankles out against the stretching strap, or belt, keeping your knees still.

Key point: This is a gentle motion. You are only trying to feel the glute contract. If you do not have a ball, substitute with a pillow.

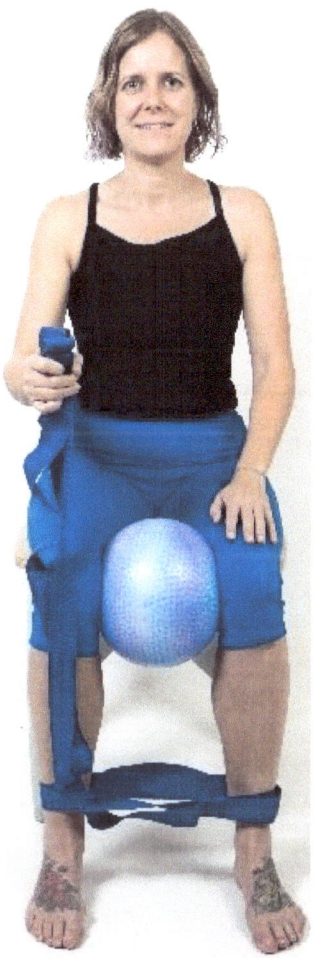

Hip External Rotators:

Reps: Start out slowly, and progress to holds from 2-10 seconds

Position: Sit on the edge of a chair, with your legs over the edge. Loop a stretching strap or belt around your thighs, keep your knees bent at a right angle. Put a ball or pillow between your ankles.

Movement: Pull thighs out against the stretching strap, or belt, keeping your ankles still.

Key point: This is a gentle motion. You are only trying to feel your glute contract.

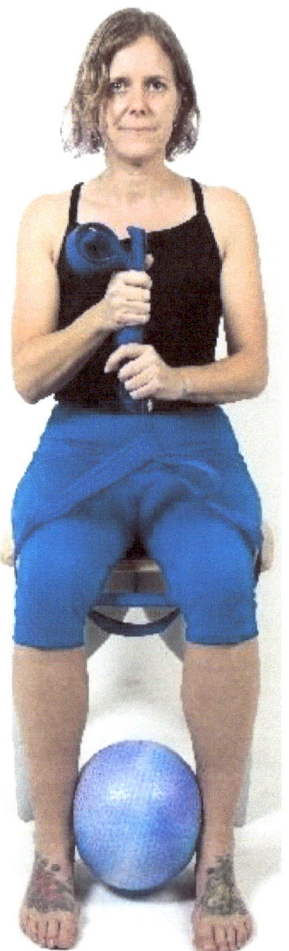

Isometric Hip Abduction with Bridging

Reps: Start with slow repetitions, and progress to holds for 3-5 seconds

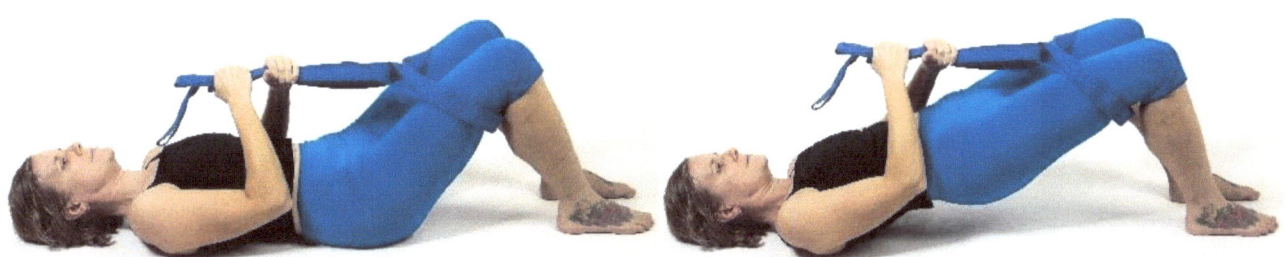

Position: Lay on your back, with your knees bent, and your feet resting on the floor. Use a stretching strap, or Pilates ring, as a form of resistance. Put the strap around your thigh, just above your knees. Walk your feet back as close to your buttocks as you can. Place your hands on your side to give you more support.

Movement: While maintaining this contraction (outer push with your thighs), raise your hips toward the ceiling. As you do this, make sure to tilt your pelvis, and pull your belly button toward your spine, to engage your transverse abdominals. Press your feet into the floor, and lift your hips to the ceiling, as high as is comfortable. As you rise, you should tighten your buttocks (but not too much) Return to the starting position.

Key point: Lightly engage the glute muscles but keep pelvic floor from clenching.

Hip Extension

Reps: Start slowly, 10 reps hold for 2 seconds, increasing to 10 seconds

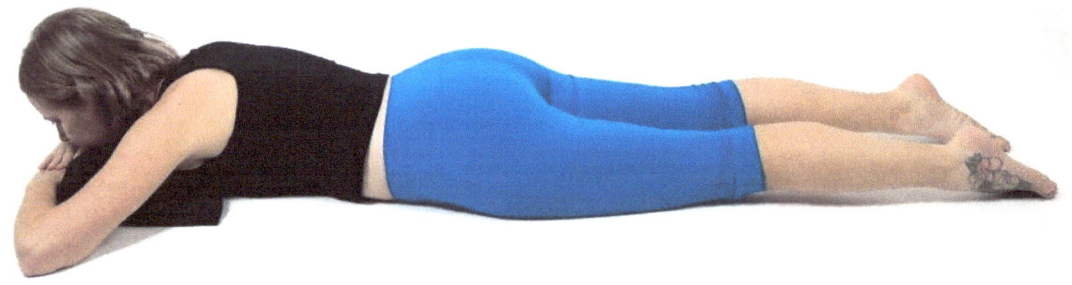

Position: Lie on your back, or stomach, with knees extended.

Movement: Tighten and maintain contraction of gluteal muscles for a 5 second hold; relaxing between each rep.

Key Point: When fully relaxed between sets, make sure you are not clenching.

Standing Hip Extension

Reps: Start slowly, 10 reps hold for 2 seconds, increasing to 10 seconds

Position: Stand on both feet

Movement: Contract core and glute muscles, kick one leg behind. Important - maintain an upright stance, with no trunk lean, and keep pelvic height even.

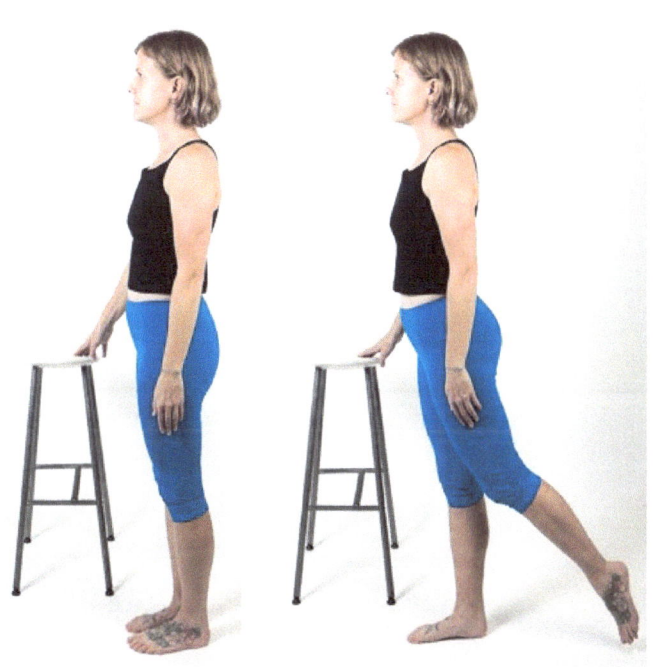

Downward Dog

Reps: Start slowly, breathe 4-8 breaths. Work up to holding the pose for 30-60 seconds

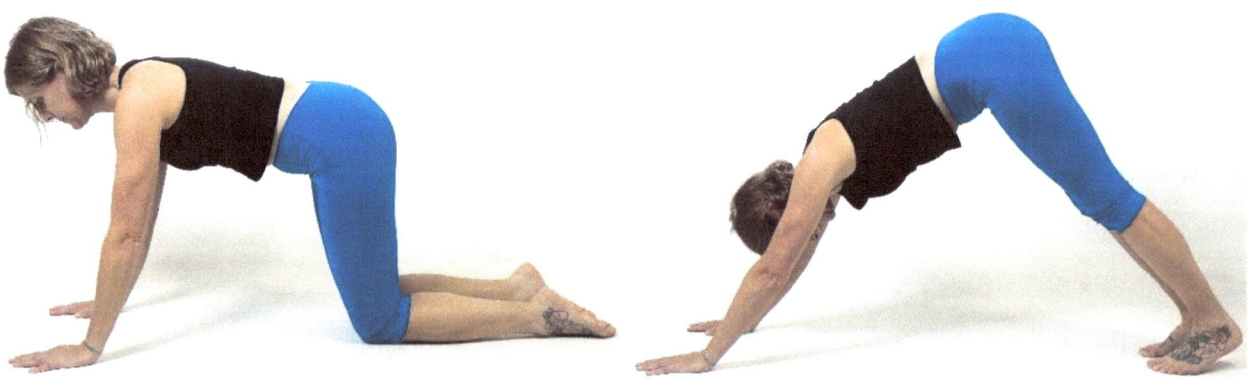

Position: Come onto the floor on your hands and knees. Set your knees directly below your hips and your hands slightly forward from your shoulders. Spread your palms, index fingers parallel or slightly turned out.

Movement: Tuck your toes under and engage your abdominal muscles as you push your body up off the floor so only your hands and feet remain on the floor. Press through your hands moving your chest gently toward your thighs and your heels gently toward the floor. You can pump each leg lightly to help release your hamstrings and calves. You will feel a stretch in your back, hamstrings, calves and ankles.

Key Point: Make sure not to clench. Focus on your pelvis remaining level. Visualize a stick balancing across your pelvis.

Calf Stretch

Reps: Start slowly, 10 reps for a total of 3 sets

Position: Stand on a step with your heels hanging off the edge. The balls of your feet should be on the step.

Movement: Holding on to a stool, very slowly, drop your heels below the level of your feet for a count of 10. Feel the stretch all the way up to your pelvis. Repeat.

Key Point: Make sure you are not clenching, keep pelvis level and do not allow it to twist.

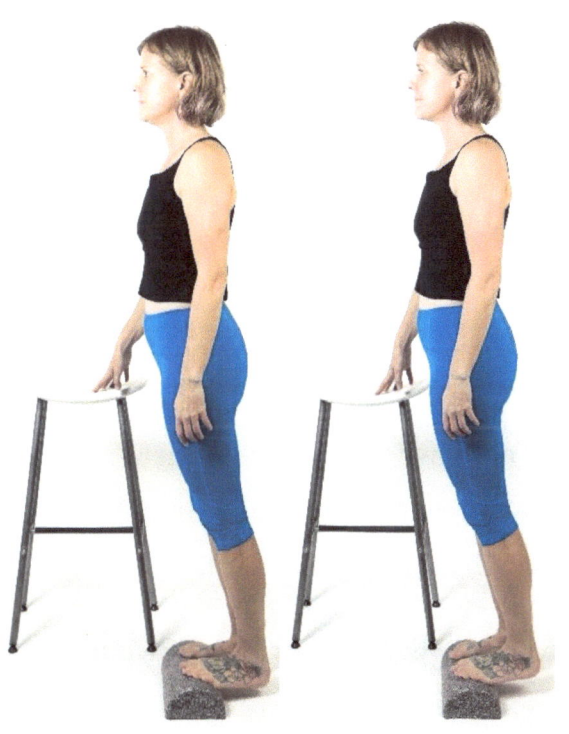

Chapter 10

Now you Know!

Living with CPP can be a thing of the past for you. As you have learned, you can be free of CPP and find true freedom from the persistent pain. You can plan to go to a movie, or on a vacation, and not have to sit close to the door of the theater or choose your vacation destination by the duration of the flight. Can you imagine a life where having pelvic pain isn't the first thing you think about when considering an activity? It is possible!

Your body heals from the inside out, and this is where the Pelvic Pain Program starts. First, we restore the floor. Then, as you achieve some relief from the pain, you learn to feel in your body exactly which muscles are involved. Once you've identified the muscles involved, you can address the poor postural patterns your body has adopted because of them. These compensatory postural patterns exacerbate CPP, causing painful and (at times) debilitating flare-ups. Finding a good chiropractor is a powerful addition to your team of practitioners to help in this area. Addressing misalignment of your pelvis and lumbar spine will help to calm down the nerves and muscles, resulting in improved function. As you progress through the Pelvic Pain Program, you will develop healthy postural patterns, thereby reducing flare-ups, and pain. I know, I have been where you are, and through my experience as a Chiropractor, extensive research, and doing exactly what I have shared here, I no longer suffer from CPP. My life, and lifestyle, has dramatically improved!

Once your posture is corrected, look at what else in your life might be exacerbating your CPP and causing flare-ups. Change those habits. Stop sitting with your legs crossed. Start using a pillow between your knees to sleep at night. Change what causes your flare-ups. Pay attention to your diet and reduce inflammatory foods. Consider some natural pain relief strategies like magnesium salts, natural pain relief supplementation, cupping, massage, and trigger point work (including dry needling). If you are close to Dr. Edward Cremata, DC, RN, in Fremont, California, he's amazing! If not, look for a qualified professional in your area who specializes in trigger points. Rebalance your core, using the breathing exercises to get your muscles working in harmony. Once you have all this, it's time to move forward with rebuilding. Incorporate the strengthening and stretching exercises, do them as I describe, and you are there! Follow the Pelvic Pain Program I have laid out and you too can be free of CPP, like me.

It is time for you to take charge of your health and your body. Act now! The longer you wait, the more issues you will have to overcome and the harder it will be. The more pain you will have, the more dysfunctional postural patterns, the more symptoms. Start now. Slowly if necessary. One day at a time move away from degeneration, and towards regeneration. You can do it, I know you can!

I will be here every step of the way. I have gone through the program myself. You will have good days and bad days. Keep the faith. Modify your hard work on bad days and take advantage of good days. You will find the good days begin to outnumber the bad days.

Yours in health,

Lavonne Pineda

Chapter 11

Bonus: Pelvic Anti-Inflammatory Diet Sample Recipes

Following a 30-day period eliminating the Top Five Inflammatory Foods (corn, soy, pork, wheat, and dairy), you can start to introduce small amounts of dairy and certain wheat products (like cracked wheat), to test your sensitivity. The goal here is to identify what foods trigger a flare-up. If you have bloating, abdominal pain, increased pelvic pain, you will need to permanently eliminate the food that affects you.

These recipes are rich in anti-inflammatory foods and have no gluten, processed sugar, or preservatives, and no pre-packaged or processed ingredients. You can try these during the 30-day elimination period.

Dinner/Lunch

Orange-Glazed Salmon with Asparagus

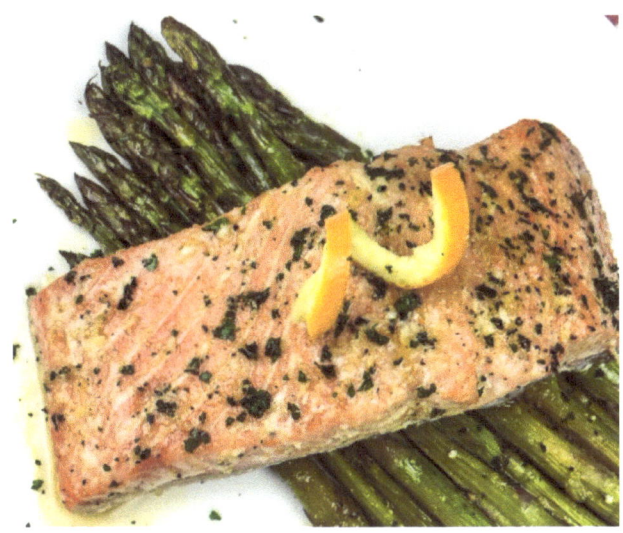

This quick and easy one pan dinner is the perfect healthy weeknight meal. From start to finish, you can have this delicious, complete meal on the table in less than 25 minutes!

Prep time: 5 minutes
Cook time: 15-18 minutes
Serves: 4

Ingredients:

4 6-oz. each salmon filets, preferably wild-caught Alaskan
3 T. fresh orange juice
2 t. honey
3 T. extra virgin olive oil
2 T. balsamic vinegar
2 garlic cloves, finely minced
1½ lb. asparagus, tough end removed
Sea salt and black pepper, to taste

Directions:

1. Preheat oven to 400°F and line a large, rimmed baking sheet with a piece of parchment paper or a Silpat® baking mat. Place the salmon fillets skin side down in the center of the baking sheet and set aside.

2. In a medium bowl, whisk together the orange juice, honey, olive oil, balsamic vinegar, and garlic. Generously season with salt and black pepper, to taste, and brush over the salmon.

3. Add the asparagus to the bowl with the orange juice mixture and gently toss to

combine. Season with additional salt and black pepper, to taste.

4. Arrange asparagus around the salmon filets in a single layer and place sheet pan in preheated oven. Bake for 15-18 minutes, or just until the salmon is flaky, and the asparagus develops a bit of color, being careful to not overcook the salmon.

5. Remove from oven and serve immediately. Enjoy!

Garlic and Chive Cauliflower Mash

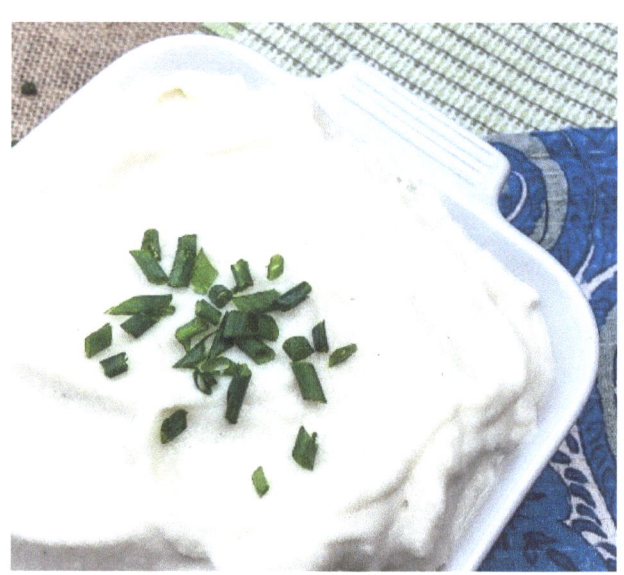

This flavorful cauliflower mash pairs well with a wide range of beef, chicken, and plant-based entrees. Plus, it comes together in under 30 minutes, so it is perfect for those busy weeknights when you want to get a healthy dinner on the table without too much fuss.

Prep time: 10 minutes
Cook time: 15 minutes
Serves: 4

Tip: Steaming the garlic along with the cauliflower will remove the raw edge and make it more tender.

Ingredients:

1 medium cauliflower head, florets only

2-3 whole garlic cloves, peeled

2 T. extra virgin olive oil

2 T. unsweetened almond milk

1 t. garlic powder

1 t. onion powder

Sea salt and black pepper, to taste

3 T. fresh chives, chopped

Directions:

1. Place the cauliflower florets and the garlic cloves into a steamer basket set over a pot of gently boiling water. Cover and steam until the cauliflower is fork-tender, around 15 minutes.

2. Transfer the cauliflower and garlic to a food processor or blender and add the olive oil, almond milk, garlic powder, and onion powder. Season with salt and black pepper, to taste, and process until smooth and creamy. Taste and adjust the seasonings, as desired.

Spicy Black Bean Taco Wraps with Fresh Guacamole

These vegetarian spicy black bean taco wraps are perfect for Meatless Mondays or anytime you want to get a plant-based meal on the table in around 20 minutes.

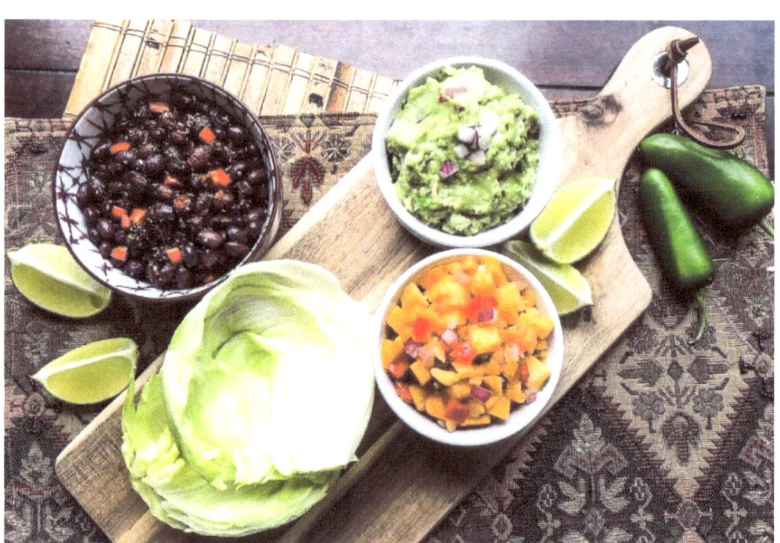

Prep time: 15 minutes
Cook time: 5 minutes
Serves: 4

Ingredients:

2 T. extra virgin olive oil
1 15-oz. can black beans, drained and rinsed
2 T. water
1 t. ground cumin
½ t. chili powder
1 t. smoked paprika
¼ t. cayenne pepper
¼ t. dried Mexican oregano
Sea salt and black pepper, to taste
Optional: ½ medium red bell pepper, finely diced

Guacamole Ingredients:

2 large ripe avocados, pitted
1 medium tomato, seeded and diced
3 T. fresh lime juice
2 T. fresh cilantro, minced
½ medium jalapeño, finely diced
Sea salt and black pepper, to taste

To Serve:

Mango Salsa*
Iceberg, butter, or Romaine lettuce leaves for wrapping

Directions:

1. Heat olive oil in a skillet over medium heat. Add beans, water, cumin, chili powder, smoked paprika, cayenne, and Mexican oregano. Season with salt and black pepper, to taste, and stir to combine.

2. Cook, stirring occasionally, until the beans are warmed through and the spices become fragrant, around 4-5 minutes. Remove from heat and set aside.

3. While the beans are cooking, mash the avocado in a small glass or other non-reactive bowl. Add tomato, lime juice, fresh cilantro, and jalapeño. Season with salt and black pepper, to taste, and stir to combine. Set aside.

4. Transfer warm beans to a bowl and add diced bell pepper, if using. Sprinkle with additional spices, if desired. Serve immediately with large lettuce leaves for wrapping, along with fresh guacamole and this spicy mango salsa. Enjoy!

Spicy Mango Salsa

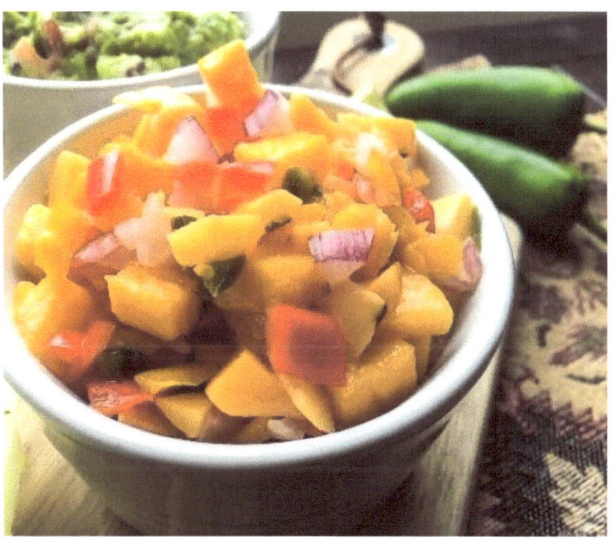

This fresh mango salsa offers a nice blend of sweet and spicy flavors. It is delicious paired with our Spicy Black Bean Taco Wraps or served on top of some grilled Atlantic cod. It also makes a fantastic snack when served with some sweet potato or even traditional tortilla chips. You'll definitely want to give this one a try!

Prep time: 10 minutes
Cook time: n/a
Serves: 4

Ingredients:

2 medium mangos, peeled and chopped small

1 medium red bell pepper, chopped small

½ medium red onion, diced small

½ medium jalapeño, finely minced

3 T. fresh cilantro, finely chopped

2 T. fresh lime juice

Sea salt and black pepper, to taste

Directions:

1. Combine mango, bell pepper, red onion, jalapeño, cilantro, and fresh lime juice in a medium glass or other non-reactive bowl. Season with salt and black pepper, to taste, and stir to combine.

2. Serve immediately or cover and place in the refrigerator until ready to use. Enjoy!

Strawberry Fennel Salad with Homemade Vinaigrette

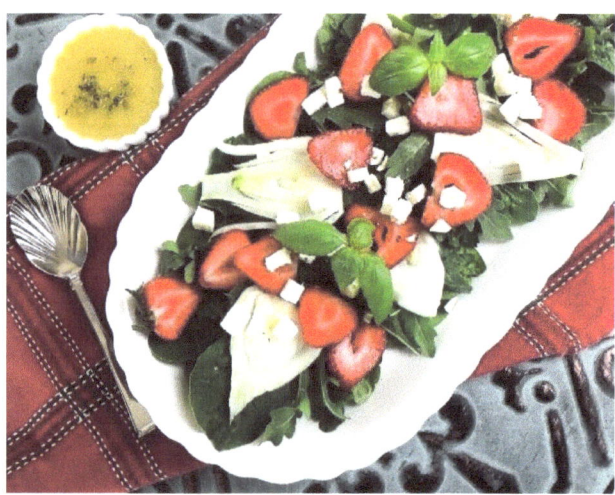

Need a quick and refreshing side dish to add a pop of color and fresh flavor to your dinner table? Look no further than this super quick and easy strawberry fennel salad. The fennel offers a satisfying crunch, while the sweet strawberries balance the natural saltiness of the Feta cheese. It comes together in just 15 minutes, so it's perfect for those busy weeknight meals.

Prep time: 15 minutes

Cook time: n/a

Serves: 4

Tip: If preferred, toss the spinach and arugula with the salad dressing prior to arranging on the platter.

Dressing Ingredients:

¼ c. extra-virgin olive oil

2 T. rice wine vinegar

1 t. Dijon mustard

½ t. Italian seasoning

Sea salt and black pepper, to taste

Salad Ingredients:

2 c. baby spinach, rinsed and patted dry

2 c. baby arugula, rinsed and patted dry

1 medium fennel bulb, trimmed and thinly sliced

1 c. strawberries, sliced

4 oz. Feta cheese, crumbled

Optional: Sprigs of fresh basil, for garnish

Directions:

1. Prepare dressing by whisking together all ingredients in a glass or other non-reactive bowl. Taste and adjust seasonings, as desired. Transfer to a serving container and set aside.

2. Arrange the spinach and arugula on a serving platter and top with sliced fennel, strawberries, and Feta cheese.

3. Serve immediately with chilled salad plates and dressing on the side. Enjoy!

Quinoa-Stuffed Butternut Squash

Prep time: 20 minutes
Cook time: 60-65 minutes
Serves: 6

Time-Saving Tip: To save time, start preparing the quinoa right after placing the butternut squash in the oven.

Ingredients:

2 medium butternut squash, cut in half lengthwise, seeds and pulp removed
1 T. extra virgin olive oil, divided
Sea salt and black pepper, to taste
1½ c. vegetable broth, preferably organic
¾ c. quinoa, uncooked
1 small bunch kale, stems removed and chopped
2-3 cloves garlic, minced
1 t. dried oregano
1 large organic orange, zest only
1 T. fresh orange juice
1/3 c. dried cranberries
½ c. Parmesan cheese, freshly grated

Directions:

1. Preheat oven to 425°F and line a large, rimmed baking sheet with parchment paper or a Silpat® baking mat.

2. Place butternut squash on prepared baking sheet, cut side up. Drizzle with 1 teaspoon olive oil and sprinkle lightly with salt and black pepper, to taste. Place baking sheet in preheated oven and roast for 45-50 minutes, or just until the squash is fork tender.

3. While the squash is roasting, pour vegetable broth into a small saucepan set over medium-high heat. Bring to a boil and add the quinoa. Return liquid to boiling, and then reduce heat to medium-low. Cover and simmer for 11-12 minutes, or until most of the broth is absorbed.

4. Remove from heat and let sit, covered, for 15 minutes. Then, fluff quinoa with a fork and set aside.

5. When the squash is ready, remove baking sheet from oven and set aside to cool. Reduce oven temperature to 375°F.

6. When the squash is cool enough to handle, scoop out the flesh, leaving a ½"-thick border around the sides and bottom. Transfer the removed fresh to a cutting board and chop into bite-sized pieces. Set aside.

7. In a large skillet, heat the remaining olive oil over medium heat. Add the kale, garlic, and oregano, and stir to combine. Season with salt and black pepper, to taste, and cook, stirring occasionally, for 4-5 minutes or just until the kale wilts.

8. Remove skillet from heat and stir in the chopped butternut squash, orange zest, orange juice, dried cranberries, and cooked quinoa. Fill each squash half with the kale-quinoa mixture, then place in the 375°F oven for 10 minutes or until warmed through.

9. Remove from oven and sprinkle with Parmesan cheese before serving. Enjoy!

Loaded Baked Potatoes with Cashew Sour Cream

Prep time: 10 minutes (+ 3 hours to soak cashews)
Cook time: 60 minutes
Serves: 6

Ingredients:

6 large Idaho potatoes, cleaned
3 c. broccoli florets, steamed and kept warm
3-4 green onions, chopped
Sea salt and black pepper, to taste
6 oz. cheddar cheese, shredded
Cashew Sour Cream:
1 c. raw cashews, soaked in water for at least 3 hours and drained
2 T. lemon juice
2 T. apple cider vinegar
2 T. cashew (or almond) milk, unsweetened
1 T. fresh dill
½ t. salt

Directions:

1. Preheat oven to 400°F and pierce each potato with a fork several times.
2. Place potatoes directly on center oven rack and bake for one hour, or until potatoes are cooked through. Remove from oven and set aside.
3. While potatoes are baking, combine the ingredients for the cashew sour cream in a high-power blender or food processor. Blend until completely smooth and creamy. Transfer to an airtight container and place in the refrigerator until ready to serve.
5. Once cool enough to handle, cut each potato in half and fluff the inside with a fork. Top each potato half with steamed broccoli and green onions. Season with salt and black pepper, to taste, and top with shredded cheddar cheese, if using.
6. Serve immediately with a generous spoonful of cashew sour cream, if desired. Enjoy!

Spinach & Arugula Cashew Salad

Prep time: 10 minutes
Cook time: n/a
Serves: 6

Ingredients:

4 c. baby spinach leaves, chopped

2 c. arugula

4 green onions, sliced thin

1 c. toasted cashews, chopped

2 T. fresh lemon juice

2 T. balsamic vinegar

½ c. extra-virgin olive oil

2 t. Dijon mustard

2 t. real maple syrup

Sea salt and black pepper, to taste

Directions:

1. Combine the spinach, arugula, green onions, and cashews in a large salad bowl. Toss gently to combine.

2. In a small bowl, combine the lemon juice, balsamic vinegar, olive oil, Dijon mustard, and maple syrup. Season with salt and black pepper, to taste, and stir to combine. Taste and adjust seasonings, as desired.

3. To serve, pour half the dressing over salad and toss to combine. Serve immediately on chilled salad plates with remaining dressing on the side. Enjoy!

Meatless Warm Nicoise Salad

Prep time: 5 minutes
Cook time: 25 minutes
Serves: 6

Ingredients:

2 T. extra virgin olive oil

1 small red onion, chopped small

12 small red potatoes, cut in half

1 12-oz. frozen green beans

2 T. water

2 t. Italian seasoning

1 t. garlic powder

Sea salt and black pepper, to taste

3 large Roma tomatoes, seeded and chopped

4 c. mixed salad greens, cleaned

3 hard-boiled eggs, chopped

Salad dressing, of choice

Directions:

1. Heat olive oil in a large skillet over medium-high heat. Add onion and sauté for 4-5 minutes, stirring frequently.

2. Add the potatoes and reduce the heat to medium-low. Cover and cook for 8-10 minutes, stirring occasionally, or until potatoes are just tender.

3. Remove lid and stir in the green beans, water, Italian seasoning, and garlic powder. Season with salt and black pepper, to taste, and stir to combine.

4. Cover and cook 6-8 minutes, stirring occasionally, or until the green beans are tender and the potatoes are golden brown.

5. Remove from heat and transfer cooked vegetables to a serving bowl filled with the chopped tomatoes and mixed salad greens. Top with chopped egg and serve immediately with favorite salad dressing. Enjoy!

Breakfast

Instant Pot Steel Cut Oats Breakfast Bowls

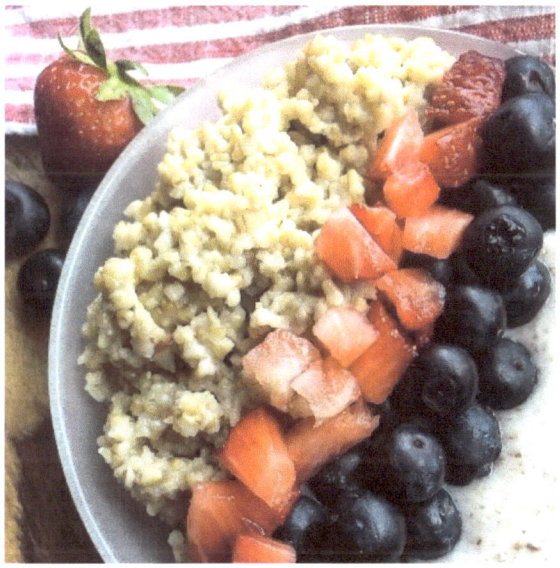

Here is a healthy and delicious breakfast idea that looks as great as it tastes! The nice thing about these Instant Pot steel cut oats is you can pretty much set it and forget it while it cooks.

Tip: To save time in the morning, prepare the yogurt mixture the night before and use blueberries and raspberries to reduce prep time.

Prep time: 10 minutes

Cook time: 25 minutes + time to come to pressure

Serves: 4

Ingredients:

Non-stick cooking spray

1 c. steel cut oats

3¼ c. water

2 c. Greek or coconut yogurt

1½ T. chia seeds

1 T. real maple syrup, plus additional for serving

1 c. fresh strawberries, hulled and cut into chunks

1 c. fresh blueberries, rinsed and patted dry

Directions:

1. Spray the Instant Pot cooking container with non-stick cooking spray.

2. Add steel cut oats and water and stir to combine. Cover with lid and lock into position, then flip the pressure valve to the "Sealing" position.

3. Press the "Manual" button and select the high heat setting. Set cook time to 10 minutes. After a brief pause, the Instant Pot will automatically start building pressure.

4. While the oats cook, combine yogurt, chia seeds, and maple syrup in a small bowl and stir to combine. Set aside.

5. When cook time is complete, turn off the Instant Pot to prevent scorching. Allow pressure to release naturally for 15 minutes, and then do a quick release for any remaining pressure.

6. Carefully remove lid and stir the contents to combine. Transfer the cooked oats to individual serving bowls. Heap the oats a little higher on one side of the bowl and spoon the yogurt mixture onto the other half. Arrange the strawberries and blueberries between the two halves for a nice presentation. Serve immediately with additional maple syrup on the side, if desired. Enjoy!

Sweet Potato and Avocado Breakfast "Toast"

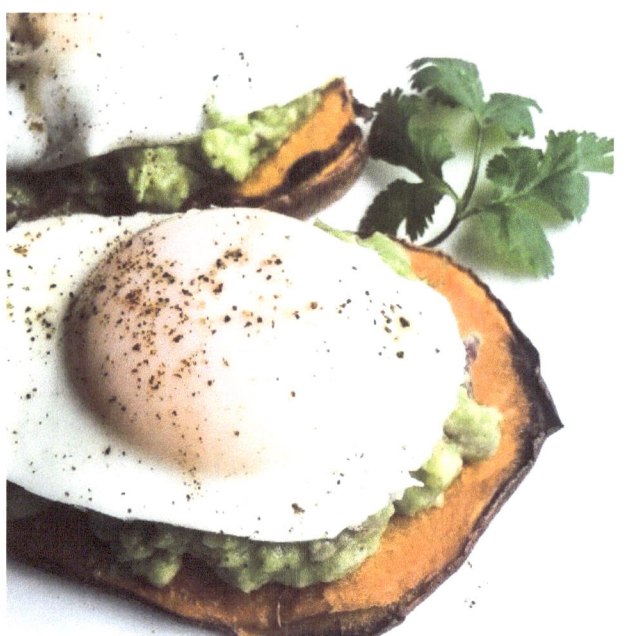

This hearty and satisfying breakfast recipe will get your day off to a great start. Although it can be prepared in 30 minutes, you can save even more time on busy weekday mornings by roasting a large batch of sliced sweet potatoes ahead of time. Simply store the pre-cooked slices in the refrigerator in an airtight container, and then pop them under the broiler or in a toaster oven to warm through before serving.

Prep time: 10 minutes
Cook time: 20 minutes
Serves: 4

Ingredients:

1-2 medium sweet potatoes, sliced ¼" thick (8 slices total)

2 T. extra virgin olive oil, divided

8 large eggs

2 ripe avocadoes

1 medium tomato, seeded and diced

½ c. fresh cilantro, chopped

3 T. fresh lime juice

1 t. red pepper flakes

Sea salt and black pepper, to taste

Optional: Smoked paprika, for garnish

Directions:

1. Preheat oven to 425°F and place a wire rack inside a large, rimmed baking sheet. Spray rack with non-stick cooking spray and set aside.

2. While the oven is heating, mash the avocados in a medium bowl with a fork. Add tomatoes, cilantro, lime juice, and red pepper flakes. Season with salt and black pepper, to taste, and stir to combine. Set aside.

3. Arrange the sweet potato slices on the prepared wire rack and place in the preheated oven for 15-20 minutes or until slices are fork tender, turning once halfway through cooking. Remove from oven and set aside.

4. While the sweet potato slices are cooking, heat half the olive oil in a large non-stick sauté pan over medium-low heat. Add 4 eggs and season with salt and black pepper, to taste.

5. Cover pan and cook until the whites are set, and the yolks are done to the desired consistency, around 3-5 minutes. Remove lid and transfer eggs to a plate and keep warm. Repeat with the remaining 4 eggs.

6. To serve, top each sweet potato slice with a spoonful of fresh guacamole and a warm sunny-side-up egg. Sprinkle with smoked paprika, if desired. Enjoy!

Mixed Berry Parfait with Warm Raspberry Sauce

Prep time: 10 minutes
Cook time: 3 minutes
Serves: 6

Ingredients:

2 c. fresh strawberries, hulled and cut into chunks
2 c. fresh blueberries
3 c. fresh raspberries, divided
2 T. water
1 T. real maple syrup
1 T. fresh lemon juice
3 T. sugar-free strawberry preserves
3 c. coconut yogurt, unsweetened
3/4 c. roasted almonds, chopped

Directions:

1. Add strawberries, blueberries, and one cup raspberries to a medium-sized bowl. Toss gently to combine.

2. Add remaining raspberries, one tablespoon water, maple syrup, and lemon juice to a food processor or blender and puree until smooth. Add additional water if mixture is too thick to pour.

3. Gently heat the strawberry preserves in a small saucepan over low heat. Stir in the raspberry puree until combined and heated through, approximately 2-3 minutes. Remove from heat and set aside.

4. To serve, divide yogurt between four chilled dessert bowls and top with fresh berries. Pour warm berry sauce over each dish and top with chopped almonds. Enjoy!

Breakfast: Cherry & Almond Granola

Serves 6
Prep time: 5 minutes + 10 minutes to cool
Cook time: 25 minutes

Ingredients:

3 c. old-fashioned rolled oats (organic), uncooked

1 c. slivered almonds

½ c. raw sunflower seeds

¼ c. coconut oil, melted

3 T. pure maple syrup

2 t. vanilla extract

½ t. sea salt

¾ c. dried cherries

¼ c. coconut flakes, finely chopped

Optional: Greek or non-dairy yogurt and seasonal berries

Directions:

1. Preheat oven to 400°F and line a large rimmed baking sheet with a piece of parchment paper. Set aside.

2. Add all ingredients, except for cherries and coconut, in a large bowl and mix until dry ingredients are lightly coated with coconut oil, maple syrup and vanilla extract.

3. Spread the granola mixture into a thin layer on the prepared baking sheet and place in the pre-heated oven for 20-25 minutes, or until granola is golden brown. While baking, stir granola every 5-6 minutes with a wooden spoon so it browns evenly.

4. Remove from oven and stir in the cherries and coconut while still warm. Allow the granola to cool down completely before serving with some Greek or non-dairy yogurt and fresh seasonal berries, if desired. Enjoy!

Blueberry Breakfast Smoothie

Prep time: 5 minutes

Cook time: n/a

Serves: 2

Ingredients:

1¾ c. almond milk, unsweetened

1½ c. fresh blueberries (can also use frozen)

½ c. coconut yogurt

1 large banana, cut in chunks and frozen

1 t. honey, preferably local

3-4 large ice cubes

Directions:

1. Add ingredients in the order listed to a high-powered blender container.

2. Blend until completely smooth and frothy.

3. Pour into chilled glasses and serve immediately. Enjoy!

Deserts

Creamy Instant Pot Rice Pudding

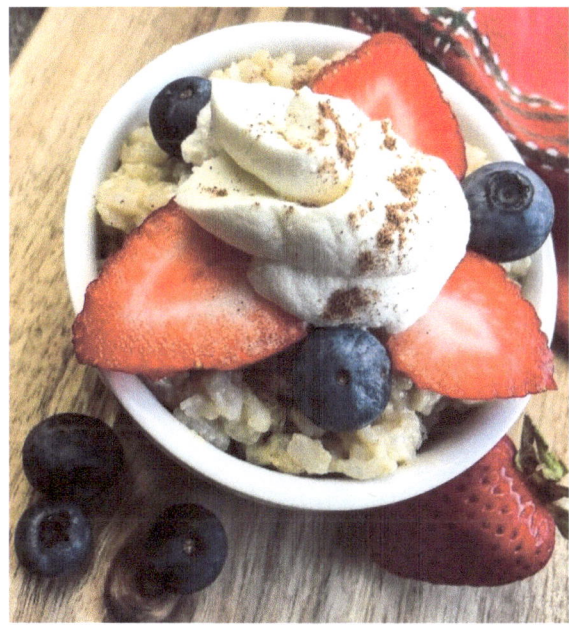

This creamy, custard-like rice pudding is so delicious and easy to make, it just might become your new favorite dessert. It is wonderful on its own with a sprinkle of ground cinnamon and maple syrup or with some fresh berries and whipped cream.

Prep time: 5 minutes

Cook time: 25 minutes + time to come to pressure

Serves: 4-6

Ingredients:

2 T. extra virgin olive oil

1 c. Arborio rice, rinsed and well drained

2½ c. almond milk, divided

2 T. maple syrup

1 t. real vanilla extract

1 t. ground cinnamon

¼ t. salt

2 eggs

Optional toppings and garnish:

Fresh berries

Whipped cream

Ground cinnamon

Real maple syrup

Cinnamon sticks

Directions:

1. Add olive oil to Instant Pot and press the "Sauté" button. Adjust heat setting to normal. Add rice and stir until coated in the

oil and lightly toasted, approximately 2 minutes.

2. Turn Instant Pot off and add 2 cups almond milk, maple syrup, vanilla extra, cinnamon, and salt. Stir to combine.

3. Add lid and lock into place. Press the "Manual" button and adjust setting to high. Set cook time to 10 minutes and set the pressure valve to "Sealing." After a brief pause, the Instant Pot will automatically start building pressure.

4. Meanwhile, whisk the eggs with the remaining almond milk in a medium-sized mixing bowl and set aside.

5. When the cook time is complete, turn the Instant Pot off to prevent scorching. Allow pressure to release naturally for 15 minutes, and then release the remaining pressure manually.

6. Unlock and remove lid and transfer one heaping spoonful of the hot rice mixture to the beaten eggs and stir to combine. Repeat with another spoonful of rice before slowly whisking the tempered egg mixture into the Instant Pot.

7. Press the "Sauté" button and adjust the heat setting to normal. Stir the mixture continually until the pudding thickens and the egg is thoroughly incorporated, approximately 3-4 minutes.

8. Turn the Instant Pot off and immediately remove the cooking container to prevent scorching. Allow pudding to cool slightly before serving or transfer to a storage container and press a layer of plastic wrap across the surface before placing in the refrigerator.

9. Serve warm or chilled topped with fresh fruit or warm berry compote and a dollop of whipped cream, if desired. Enjoy!

Chocolate Hazelnut Truffles

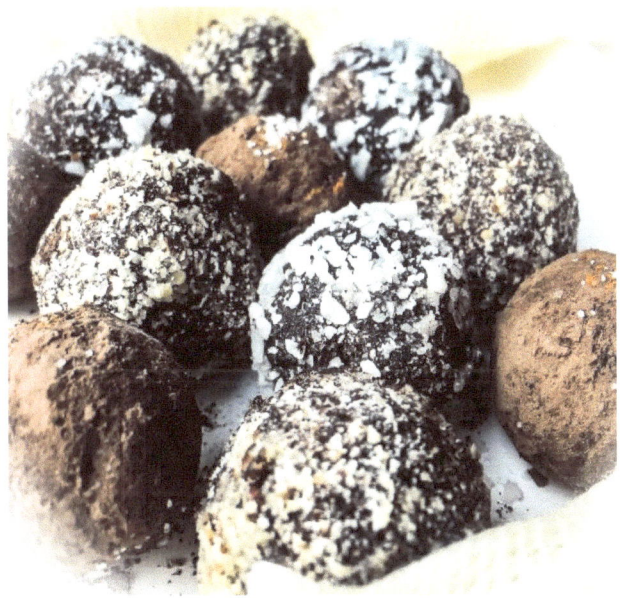

Looking for a delicious snack to satisfy your sweet tooth? Look no further than these decadent chocolate hazelnut truffles. The best part? Dates and a touch of maple syrup add just enough sweetness without adding any refined sugar.

Prep time: 25 minutes
Cook time: n/a
Yield: 15-18 truffles

Ingredients:

½ c. raw hazelnuts
12 Medjool dates, pitted
2 T. cocoa powder, unsweetened
2 T. coconut flour
1 T. coconut oil, melted
1½ T. pure maple syrup
1 t. pure vanilla extract
¼ t. coarse salt

Optional Coatings:

¼ c. hazelnuts or almonds, ground
¼ c. coconut flakes, finely shredded
2 T unsweetened cocoa powder + ¼ t. each cayenne pepper and coarse salt

Directions:

1. Place pitted dates in a small bowl filled with warm water. Set aside to soak for 10-15 minutes.

2. Line a rimmed baking sheet with wax paper and set aside. Pour each selected coating, if using, onto a separate shallow, rimmed plate and set aside.

3. Add hazelnuts to a food processor and process until finely ground.

4. Remove the softened dates from bowl and drain off any excess water. Add dates and cocoa powder to food processor and blend until smooth, approximately 3-4 minutes. Scrape the sides, as necessary, to ensure mixture is thoroughly combined.

5. Tip: Add a few drops of water at a time, if necessary, to achieve a smooth consistency, but don't add too much.

6. Add coconut flour, coconut oil, maple syrup, vanilla extract, and salt to the mixture and process until combined.

7. Remove the dough from the food processor and divide into 15-18 equal-sized portions. Roll each section of dough into a ball before rolling in the selected coatings.

8. Once coated, place on prepared baking tray and place in the refrigerator to chill for several minutes before serving. Enjoy!

Stuffed Pineapple Fruit Salad

Serves 4
Prep time: 30 minutes
Cook time: n/a

Dressing Ingredients:

¼ c. orange juice
2 t. orange zest
2 T. lemon juice
2 t. lemon zest
1/3 c. extra virgin olive oil
2 T. honey, preferably local
1 t. Dijon mustard
Sea salt and black pepper, to taste

Salad Ingredients:

2 whole pineapples
2 c. fresh mango, diced
2 c. fresh strawberries, washed, and cut in half
1 c. green grapes, cut in half
1 c. fresh blueberries
¼ c. fresh mint, chopped

Directions:

1. Prepare the dressing by combining all ingredients in a glass or other non-reactive bowl and whisk thoroughly to combine. Add salt and pepper, to taste, and set aside.

2. Cut both pineapples in half from crown to bottom with a large, sharp knife. Cut through the leafy crown so it is still attached to each half.

3. Cut around the inside edge of the pineapple with a small knife, leaving about ½" around the outside wall. Score the pineapple flesh with the knife horizontally and vertically to create a series of square sections. Scoop out the pineapple squares and transfer them to a bowl. Remove all remaining pineapple flesh until the remaining skin forms a hollowed out bowl. Repeat this process with remaining 3 pineapple halves.

4. In a separate bowl, combine the fresh pineapple chunks with the mango, strawberries, grapes, blueberries, and fresh mint. Toss gently with half the dressing and divide among the four empty pineapple shells.

5. Serve immediately with the remaining dressing on the side. Enjoy!

Frozen Watermelon-Mint Slushies

Prep time: 10 minutes
Cook time: n/a
Serves: 6

Ingredients:
6 c. fresh watermelon, seeds removed and cut into chunks
3 medium limes, juiced
1 T. honey, preferably local*
5-6 fresh mint leaves
6-8 large ice cubes

*Use more or less honey to reach desired level of sweetness.

Optional garnish: 6 fresh mint sprigs

Directions:
1. Combine all ingredients, except the mint sprigs, in a high-powered blender and blend until thoroughly combined.
2. To serve, pour into chilled serving glasses and garnish each with a sprig of fresh mint, if using. Enjoy!

Bibliography

Cell Reports. (2016, June 7). Diet mimicking fasting promotes regeneration and reduces autoimmunity and multiple sclerosis symptoms. *Reports, 15*(10), 2136-2146. Retrieved from https://www.ncbi.nlm.nih.gov/pmc/articles/PMC4899145/

Cremata DC RN, E. (2018, November 1). DC RN. (L. C. Pineda, Interviewer) Fremont, CA, USA.

de Punder, K., & Pruimboom, L. (2013). The Dietary Intake of Wheat and Other Cereal Grains and Their Role in Inflammation. *Nutrients, 5*(3), 771-787. Retrieved from https://www.ncbi.nlm.nih.gov/pmc/articles/PMC3705319/

Dommerholt, J. (2011, November). Dry needling - Peripheral and central considerations. *The Journal of Manual and Manipulative Therapy, 19*(4), 223-7. Retrieved from https://www.ncbi.nlm.nih.gov/pmc/articles/PMC3201653/

Faris, M. A., Kacimi, S., Al-Kurd, R. A., Fararieh, M. A., Mohammad, M. K., Salem, M. L., & Bustanji, Y. K. (2012, December). Intermittent fasting during Ramadan attenuates proinflammatory cytokines and immune cells in healthy subjects. *Nutrition Research, 32*(12), pp. 947-955. Retrieved from https://www.ncbi.nlm.nih.gov/pubmed/23244540

J Natl Cancer Inst. (2003, June 18). Soy, isoflavones, and breast cancer risk in Japan. *95*(12), 906-13. Retrieved from https://www.ncbi.nlm.nih.gov/pubmed/12813174

Jamieson, D. J., & Steege, J. F. (1996, January). The prevalence of dysmenorrhea, dyspareunia, pelvic pain, and irritable bowel syndrome in primary care practices. *Obstetrics Gynecology, 87*(1), 55-8.

Kelly, M. (2012, December 30). *Top 7 Genetically Modified Crops*. Retrieved from HuffPost: https://www.huffingtonpost.com/margie-kelly/genetically-modified-food_b_2039455.html

Mathias, S. D., Kuppermann, M., Liberman, R. F., Lipschutz, R. C., & Steege, J. F. (1996, March). Chronic Pelvic Pain: prevalence, health-related quality of life, and economic correlates. *Obstetrics Gynecology, 87*(3), 321-7.

Mattar, R., de Campos Mazo, D. F., & Carrilho, F. J. (2012). Lactose intolerance: diagnosis, genetic, and clinical factors. *Clinical and Experimental Gastroenterology, 5*, 113-121. Retrieved from https://www.ncbi.nlm.nih.gov/pmc/articles/PMC3401057/

Pediatrics. (2018). *Corn-Free Diet - Confectioners' Sugar Substitute*. Retrieved from UR Medicine Golisano Children's Hospital: https://www.urmc.rochester.edu/childrens-hospital/nutrition/corn-free.aspx

Reiter, R. C. (1990, March). A profile of women with chronic pelvic pain. *Clinical Obstetrics Gynocology, 33*(1), 130-6.

Singh, MD, M. K. (2018, Febuary 28). *Chronic Pelvic pain in women: History*. (E. R. Michel, Ed.) Retrieved from Medscape: https://emedicine.medscape.com/article/258334emedicine.medscape

Travell, J. G., & Simons, D. G. (1992). *Myofascial Pain and Dysfunction*. (Vol. 2). Williams & Wilkins.

Universal Health Institute. (n.d.). About Epsom Salts (MgSO4·7H2O). Chicago, IL, USA. Retrieved 2018, from Universal Health Institute: https://www.epsomsaltcouncil.org/wp-content/uploads/2015/10/universal_health_institute_about_epsom_salt.pdf

Waring, Dr R H. (2015). Report on Absorption of magnesium sulfate (Epsom salts) across the skin. University of Birmingham, UK. Retrieved from https://www.epsomsaltcouncil.org/wp-content/uploads/2015/10/report_on_absorption_of_magnesium_sulfate.pdf

NOTES:

NOTES:

NOTES:

NOTES:

www.ingramcontent.com/pod-product-compliance
Lightning Source LLC
Chambersburg PA
CBHW051911210526
45473CB00006B/1972